Health for Teens

Editor: Danielle Lobban

Volume 467

independence
educational publishers

First published by

Independence Educational Publishers
The Studio, High Green
Great Shelford
Cambridge CB22 5EG
England

www.independence.co.uk

ISBN-13: 978 1 86168 927 6

Printed in Great Britain

Printed and bound by the Pureprint Group using its environmental print technology, a low-carbon, low-waste independently audited process that reduces environmental impact using 100% renewable energy, vegetable-oil-based inks and no industrial alcohol. 98% of all dry waste and 95% of press cleaning solvents are recycled. Pureprint are ISO 14001, EMAS and FSC certified and holds the Queen's Award for Enterprise: Sustainable Development.

EU Authorised Representative: Easy Access System Europe – Mustamäe tee 50, 10621 Tallinn, Estonia
Web: www.easproject.com Email: gpsr.requests@easproject.com

MIX
Paper | Supporting responsible forestry
FSC® C022913

Acknowledgements

The publisher is grateful for permission to reproduce the material in this book. While every care has been taken to trace and acknowledge copyright, the publisher tenders its apology for any accidental infringement or where copyright has proved untraceable. The publisher would be pleased to come to a suitable arrangement in any such case with the rightful owner.

The material reproduced in **issues** books is provided as an educational resource only. The views, opinions and information contained within reprinted material in **issues** books do not necessarily represent those of Independence Educational Publishers and its employees.

Although every effort has been made to ensure that website addresses are correct at time of going to press, Independence Educational Publishers cannot be held responsible for the content of any website mentioned in this book.

Images

Cover image courtesy of Freepik. All other images courtesy of Freepik, Pixabay, Pexels, and Unsplash.

Additional acknowledgements

With thanks to the Independence team: Janey Hills, Klaudia Sommer and Jackie Staines.

Danielle Lobban

Cambridge, September 2025

Contents

Chapter 1: Looking After Your Body

Chapter 2: Protect & Prevent

Chapter 3: Looking After Your Mind

Introduction

Health for Teens is volume 467 in the **issues** series. The aim of the series is to offer current, diverse information about important issues in our world, from a UK perspective.

About *Health for Teens*

Almost 18% of the UK population are adolescents – so good health really matters. *Health for Teens* empowers you to manage stress, practise self-care, make confident health decisions, and navigate physical and mental wellbeing with ease and knowledge.

Our sources

Titles in the **issues** series are designed to function as educational resource books, providing a balanced overview of a specific subject.

The information in our books is comprised of facts, articles and opinions from many different sources, including:

- Newspaper reports and opinion pieces
- Website factsheets
- Magazine and journal articles
- Statistics and surveys
- Government reports
- Literature from special interest groups.

A note on critical evaluation

Because the information reprinted here is from a number of different sources, readers should bear in mind the origin of the text and whether the source is likely to have a particular bias when presenting information (or when conducting their research). It is hoped that, as you read about the many aspects of the issues explored in this book, you will critically evaluate the information presented.

It is important that you decide whether you are being presented with facts or opinions. Does the writer give a biased or unbiased report? If an opinion is being expressed, do you agree with the writer? Is there potential bias to the 'facts' or statistics behind an article?

Activities

Throughout this book, you will find a selection of assignments and activities designed to help you engage with the articles you have been reading and to explore your own opinions. Some tasks will take longer than others and there is a mixture of design, writing and research-based activities that you can complete alone or in a group.

Further research

At the end of each article we have listed its source and a website that you can visit if you would like to conduct your own research. Please remember to critically evaluate any sources that you consult and consider whether the information you are viewing is accurate and unbiased.

Issues Online

The **issues** series of books is complemented by our onlin resource, Issues Online.

On the Issues Online website you will find a wealth o information, covering over 75 topics, to support the PSH and RSE curriculum.

Why Issues Online?

Researching a topic? Issues Online is the best place to star for...

Librarians

Issues Online is an essential tool for librarians: feel confiden you are signposting safe, reliable, user-friendly onlin resources to students and teaching staff alike. We provid multi-user concurrent access, so no waiting around fo another student to finish with a resource. Issues Online als provides FREE downloadable posters for your shelf/wal table displays.

Teachers

Issues Online is an ideal resource for lesson plannin inspiring lively debate in class, and setting lessons an homework tasks.

Our accessible, engaging content helps deepen student knowledge, promotes critical thinking, and develop independent learning skills.

Issues Online saves precious preparation time. We wad through the wealth of material on the internet to filter th best quality, most relevant and up-to-date information yo need to start exploring a topic.

Our carefully selected, balanced content presents a overview and insight into each topic from a variety c sources and viewpoints.

Students

Issues Online is designed to support your studies in a broa range of topics, particularly social issues relevant to youn people today.

There are thousands of articles, statistics and infograph instantly available to help you with homework, researc and assignments.

With 24/7 access using the powerful Algolia search systen you can find relevant information quickly, easily and safel anytime from your laptop, tablet or smartphone, in class c at home.

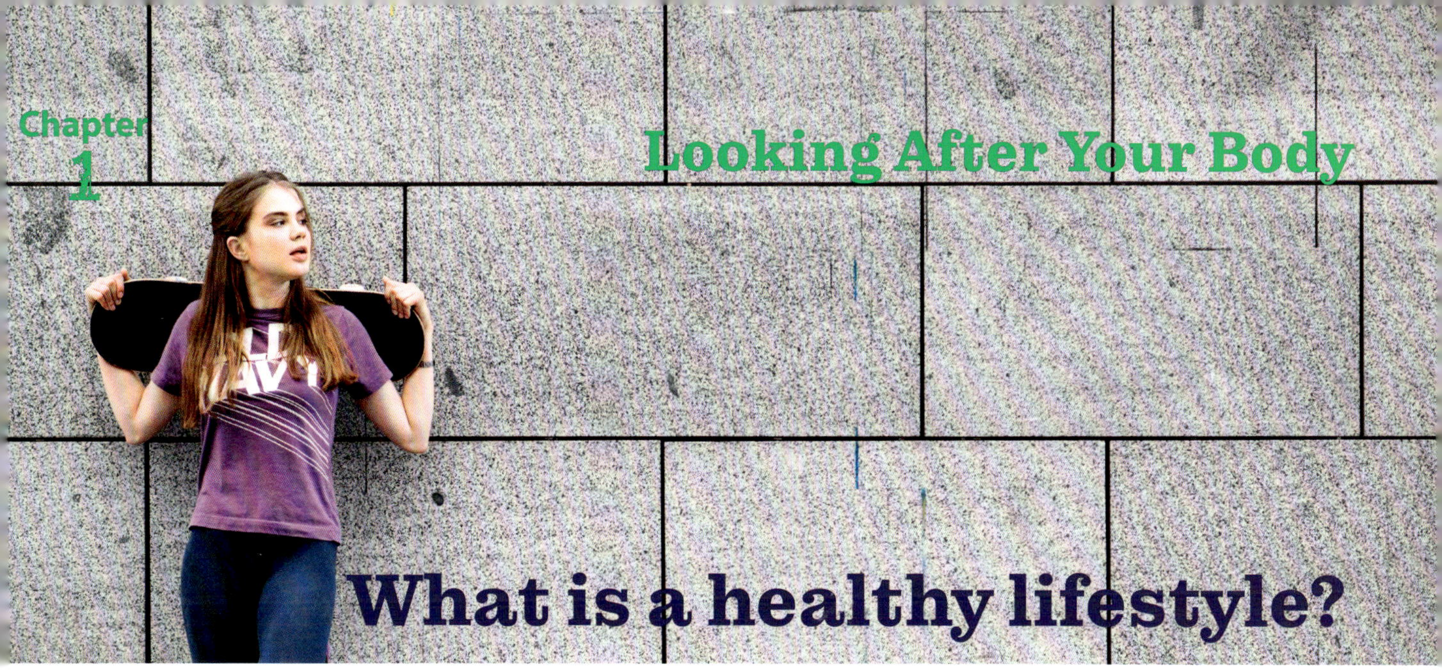

Chapter 1

Looking After Your Body

What is a healthy lifestyle?

magine sitting in class after only four hours of sleep – struggling to focus, yawning constantly and wishing you had more energy. For many teenagers, this is a common xperience. A healthier lifestyle means looking after your ody, mind and social wellbeing in ways that suit your stage f life. This article explores what a healthier lifestyle looks ke, how to maintain physical health, how to balance your aily routine, ways to care for your mental wellbeing, and ow to take charge of important health choices.

What does a 'healthier lifestyle' look like?

healthier lifestyle is about more than eating salad or going or a run. It includes physical health, mental wellbeing and ocial connections. Daily habits like getting enough sleep, miting screen time and staying hydrated make a big ifference. The benefits include higher energy levels, better oncentration in school, improved mood and greater self-onfidence.

Maintaining physical health

ood choices

Vhat you eat fuels your body and mind. Choosing holefoods – such as fruits, vegetables, whole grains and an proteins – provides long-lasting energy. Try to cut back n processed snacks, sugary drinks and too much fast food. simple swap, like sparkling water instead of fizzy soda, can nake a real difference.

hysical activity

ovement is vital for teenage health. Aim for at least 60 inutes of activity each day, from sports clubs to brisk alks. Mix up your routine with strength, flexibility and ardio exercises. Fun options like dance classes, swimming, r cycling with friends keep fitness enjoyable while building sting habits.

alanced lifestyle

ood health means more than diet and exercise. Learning balance schoolwork, hobbies and rest is key. Aim for 8–10 ours of sleep each night to recharge your body and brain. cheduling regular breaks, down-time and social activities elps prevent burnout and keeps life in balance.

Looking after mental health

Teenagers often face pressure from exams, friendships and the constant presence of social media. Recognising these stressors is the first step. Healthy coping strategies include mindfulness, deep breathing, journaling or talking to someone you trust. Building resilience can be as simple as setting realistic goals and celebrating small achievements. Sometimes professional support is needed – a school counsellor, helpline or mental-health app can provide guidance. Taking care of your mental health is just as important as looking after your body.

Taking charge of your health choices

Taking responsibility for your health

Being responsible for your own health also means knowing when to ask for help. If something doesn't feel right, don't be afraid to book an appointment with your GP or talk to a nurse. Health professionals are there to listen and support you – no problem is too small to discuss. It's also important to rely on trusted sources of information, such as the NHS website or school health services, rather than rumours or unverified social media posts. Taking these steps shows maturity and helps you make informed decisions about your wellbeing.

Vaccinations

Staying up to date with vaccinations protects you and others. Teenagers may be offered key immunisations like the HPV vaccine, meningitis protection and booster shots. These are usually given through school clinics or at your GP surgery. Remember – you have the right to ask questions and give consent for your care.

Blood and organ donation

When you reach the eligible age, donating blood is a safe and generous way to help others. Organ donation decisions can be registered through the NHS or linked to your driving licence. Choosing to donate is a powerful act of kindness with long-term impact.

How clean are Brits? New YouGov survey reveals hygiene habits

By Janice Fernandes

Hygiene habits in the UK

How often, if at all, do you do the following activities? (% of UK adults)

	More than once a day	Once a day	4 to 6 times a week	2 to 3 times a week	Once a week	Once every 2 to 3 weeks	Once a month	Less often than once a month	Never	Don't know
Brush teeth	72	23	2	1	0	0	0	0	0	1
Floss or use interdental brushes	10	25	8	10	7	4	4	9	20	3
Shower or bathe	9	46	18	20	3	1	0	1	0	1
Wash hair	2	23	15	40	13	3	1	2	2	1
Clean under fingernails	14	29	13	15	10	4	2	4	5	5
Change bed linens	0	1	1	4	39	37	11	5	0	2
Disinfect frequently touched surfaces at home/work	14	20	11	16	16	5	3	6	5	4
Clean your mobile phone screen, laptop screen, etc.	5	9	6	13	20	12	11	16	4	4
Change towels	1	6	6	21	44	13	5	2	0	2
Apply deodorant	20	59	5	5	2	1	1	2	5	1
Clean your toilet	5	15	10	25	30	8	3	1	1	3

Source: YouGov

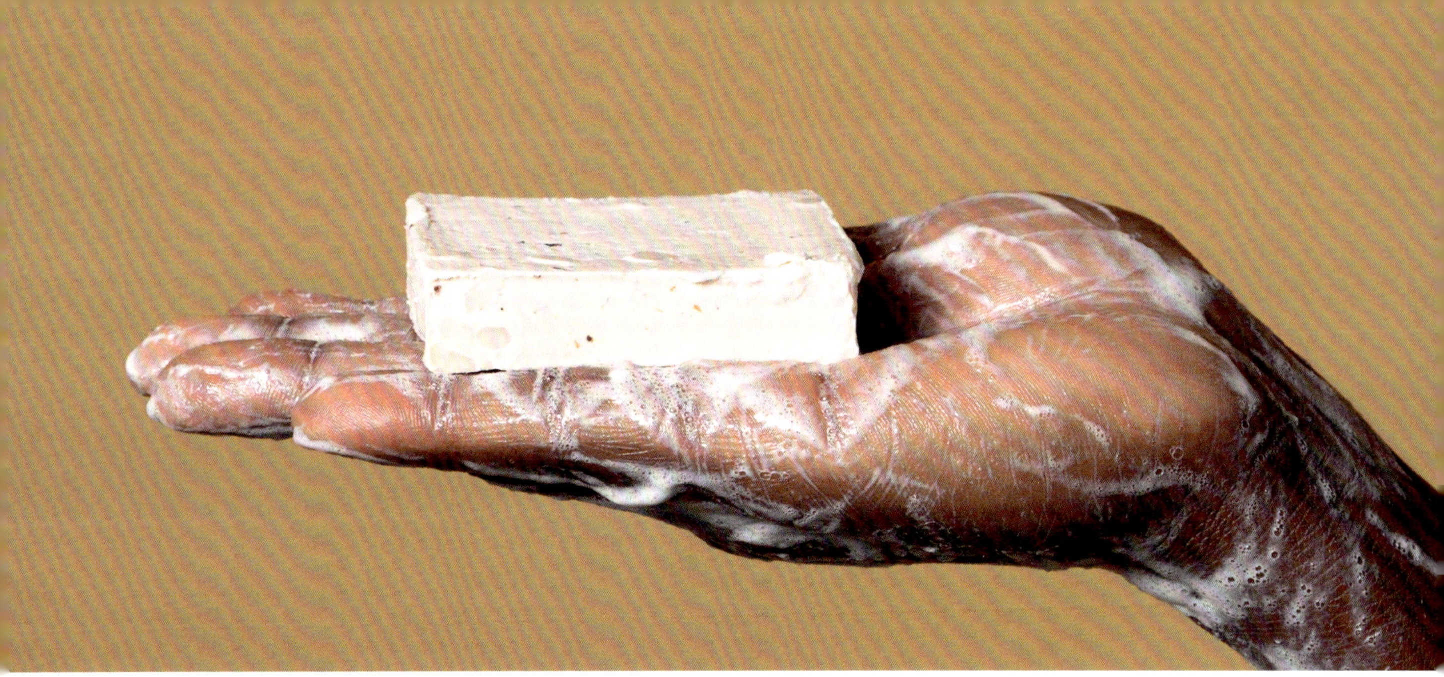

Earlier this year, the NHS issued warnings about rising flu cases, bringing renewed attention to the importance of hand hygiene and surface cleanliness. Against this ɔackdrop, a new YouGov Surveys: Serviced poll looks at how ɔften adults in the UK follow everyday hygiene routines. ·rom brushing teeth and showering to disinfecting phones ınd using hand sanitiser, the findings highlight which habits ıre widely practiced, which are often overlooked, and where :lear differences appear between men and women.

Toothbrushing is consistent – but flossing is far less common

3rushing teeth is one of the most widely maintained hygiene outines across the population. Nearly three-quarters of JK adults (72%) say they brush more than once a day, and ınother 23% brush once daily. However, a gender divide ıppears here: women are more likely than men to brush nore than once daily (79% vs. 65%), with men slightly more ikely to brush only once (28%).

lossing, on the other hand, is less embedded in daily outines. Around 35% of adults floss at least once a day, and ne in five (20%) say they never do. Men are more likely than vomen to skip flossing altogether (25% vs. 16%).

›howering, hair washing, and grooming show strong habits – but also gender contrasts

Iearly half (46%) of UK adults shower or bathe daily, and this gure is consistent between men and women. However, hair vashing shows a stronger split. While 34% of men wash their ıair every day, only 13% of women do the same. The most ommon routine among women is washing two to three imes a week (50%), compared to 30% of men – showing a lifferent approach to haircare.

:leaning under fingernails is a habit that varies widely. Just nder a third (29%) of all adults say they do this once a day, 3% say 4–6 times a week, and another 15% say 2–3 times week.

Vomen are much more likely than men to clean under their ngernails once a day (36% vs. 22%). Men are also more kely to say they never clean under their nails (7% vs. 3%).

his gap is similar across several other categories. For xample, 64% of women apply deodorant once a day compared to 55% of men, and 22% of women do so more than once daily versus 18% of men.

Hand hygiene holds strong after the toilet, but drops before meals

The majority of UK adults (82%) say they always wash their hands after using the toilet – slightly higher among women (85%) than men (78%). Handwashing before meals, however, sees a drop-off: only 36% say they always wash their hands before eating, and nearly a quarter (24%) say they only sometimes do. Here, men and women are more closely aligned.

When soap isn't available, one in three adults (34%) always use hand sanitiser. But again, women show more consistent behaviour, with 40% always using it compared to 28% of men.

Cleaning habits around the home show uneven frequency

Household hygiene habits are more variable. When it comes to disinfecting frequently touched surfaces, 34% of adults say they do this once a day or more.

Toilet cleaning is a standard practice among all. Weekly cleaning is the most common (30%), with little differences between women and men.

Device cleaning is a low-priority task for many. Only 14% of adults clean their phone, laptops, or other device screens daily, and around one in six (16%) say they do so less than once a month.

Laundry habits are mostly consistent – but bed linen changes vary

Towel-changing is fairly regular, with 44% doing so weekly and another 21% doing so multiple times per week. Bed linens are less frequently changed: 39% of adults say they change their sheets weekly, while 37% do so every two to three weeks.

14 April 2025

www.yougov.co.uk

Personal hygiene checklist

It's important for your body to stay clean and healthy.

Particularly as you grow through puberty. During this time your body will begin to sweat more, your skin and hair may become greasier, plus hair will start to grow in new places.

There's no need to be overwhelmed though, here's a checklist for keeping on top of your personal hygiene.

1. Cleaning your teeth – once in the morning and once at night before bed

We don't just brush our teeth to have fresh breath. Having good oral health prevents cavities or plaque from building up and results in a healthy smile.

You can also use floss to get rid of plaque in between teeth.

2. Cleaning genitals

Make cleaning your genitals a habit. During puberty you may start to notice discharge from this area, which is normal, but if it begins to change colour, smell or itch then speak to a GP. This can be a sign of infection.

For boys:

Gently clean underneath the foreskin everyday when washing the rest of your body. Without regular cleaning, a build-up of a whitish-yellow substance known as 'smegma' can occur under the foreskin.

Smegma can look like pus to the untrained eye. If you have any concerns consult your GP.

For girls:

Avoid using fragranced products to clean the vagina. Products that are fragranced can affect your pH levels and cause irritation.

The vagina is really good at cleaning itself. You should still clean it regularly, but when cleaning use plain, unfragranced products.

Avoid douches too – douches flush water up into the vagina. Some people use this technique thinking that it will 'cleanse' the vagina, whereas it can actually disrupt your natural pH levels.

There is no evidence that douching protects against STI's or infections either.

3. Take a shower or bath once a day

This eliminates body odour; it'll make you smell nice too. Wash your whole body and address any breakouts of spots with mild face wash.

When washing your hair:

- Be sure to massage the shampoo into the scalp. If you're using conditioner, focus it mostly on the ends of your hair, as too much conditioner can result in hair still looking wet/dirty.
- Once you've applied shampoo and conditioner, rinse it off thoroughly to remove any excess product.
- If you don't rinse your hair thoroughly, hair products can build up on your hair or scalp. This could later result in dandruff or itchiness

4. Shaving your face

Ensure you exfoliate before shaving as this will remove dead skin and gives better results. Potentially preventing 'shavers' rash' or skin irritation.

Replacing your razor blade every 7 days will prevent any skin infections from occurring.

Remember to ask for help if you need it. You may need supervision from a parent or carer at first for some support.

5. Applying deodorant

Use antiperspirant under your armpits once a day, or after any intense physical activity.

This will limit perspiration (sweating) and help to reduce body odour.

Top tip:

Some deodorants, such as body spray, do not prevent sweating. Make sure you use an antiperspirant deodorant under your arms, and not body spray.

6. Diet

A balanced diet is important for:

- Boosting mood
- Providing the body with vitamins and nutrients that we may lack
- Healthy skin

7. Exercise

Exercise can make you sweat, which is good for the body. Sweating releases toxins, boosting the immune system. Just make sure you wash your body and apply antiperspirant after any intense exercise or sweating, as dry sweat can lead to body odour.

8. Maintaining healthy nails

Keep your finger and toenails at a manageable length, clipping and cleaning them when they look long or dirty.

8 March 2023

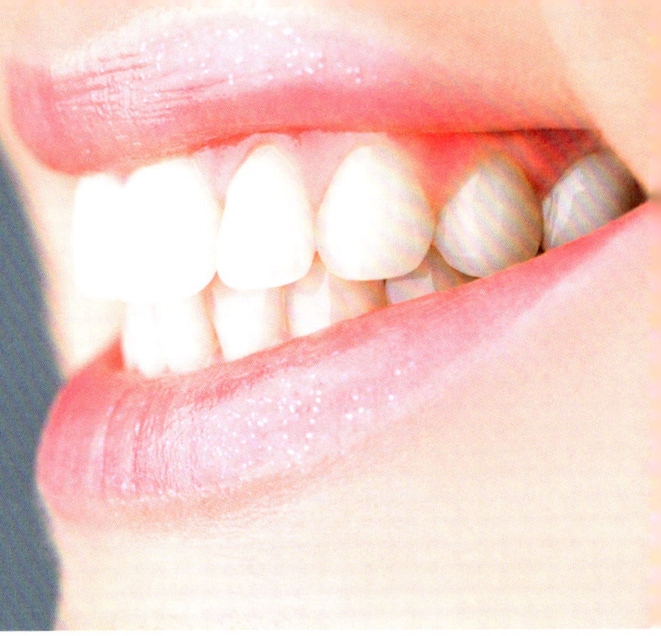

A healthy mouth – more than just a smile

eeth and gums do more than enable chewing, speaking, nd smiling. They are an important part of overall vellbeing, and taking care of them can bring benefits ar beyond the mouth.

A confident smile can shape first impressions, influence relationships, and boost self-esteem. Good oral health has also been linked with better eneral health, and growing research is helping to explain he connections between the mouth and the rest of the ody.

Keeping natural teeth for life

rushing twice daily with fluoride toothpaste, eating a alanced, low-sugar diet, and attending regular dental heck-ups can greatly reduce the risk of tooth decay and um disease – the two leading causes of tooth loss.

tudies have shown a link between the number of natural eeth retained in later life and longevity. For example, eople with 20 or more teeth at the age of 70 were found to ave a better chance of living longer than those with fewer. Vhile tooth count is not the only factor, it can reflect lifelong ealth habits and access to care.

The mouth–body connection

he mouth hosts millions of bacteria, many of them armless. When gum disease develops, harmful bacteria an enter the bloodstream. This may trigger inflammation, vhich in turn has been linked with a higher risk of certain ealth problems.

or instance, gum disease is associated with an increased kelihood of heart disease and stroke. Scientists suggest hat bacteria or the body's inflammatory response could be nvolved, although shared risk factors such as smoking, poor iet, and limited access to healthcare may also play a role.

here is also a recognised two-way relationship between um disease and type 2 diabetes. Diabetes can worsen gum roblems, and gum disease may make blood sugar more ifficult to control.

Gum health and healthy ageing

vidence suggests that poor gum health may be linked o an earlier onset of frailty, including conditions such as ementia.

While more research is needed to fully understand the connection, maintaining healthy gums appears to be one of several factors that support healthier ageing.

Pregnancy and oral health

Some studies have explored whether gum disease during pregnancy could be linked with premature birth or low birth weight.

Some research indicates that women with gum disease are more likely to give birth early, possibly due to the body's inflammatory response. Results, however, remain mixed, and more high-quality studies are needed.

What is clear is that maintaining good oral health during pregnancy is safe, beneficial, and supports the wellbeing of both mother and baby.

Looking after appearance and freshness

Healthy teeth and gums also help prevent bad breath, often caused by a build-up of plaque. Consistent daily cleaning and regular dental visits are key to avoiding this problem.

Tooth staining – from tea, coffee, red wine, or smoking – is common and usually harmless, though it can affect confidence in a smile. Brushing well can help prevent some staining, and a dental professional can remove more stubborn marks.

The take-home message

Good oral health is part of good general health. While the precise ways in which the mouth and body influence each other are still being investigated, the evidence strongly supports the importance of a healthy mouth in maintaining overall wellbeing. Brushing twice a day, limiting sugary foods and drinks, and attending dental check-ups regularly gives both the smile and the body the best chance to stay healthy.

The above information is reprinted with kind permission from Oral Health Foundation.

www.dentalhealth.org

Teens' teeth

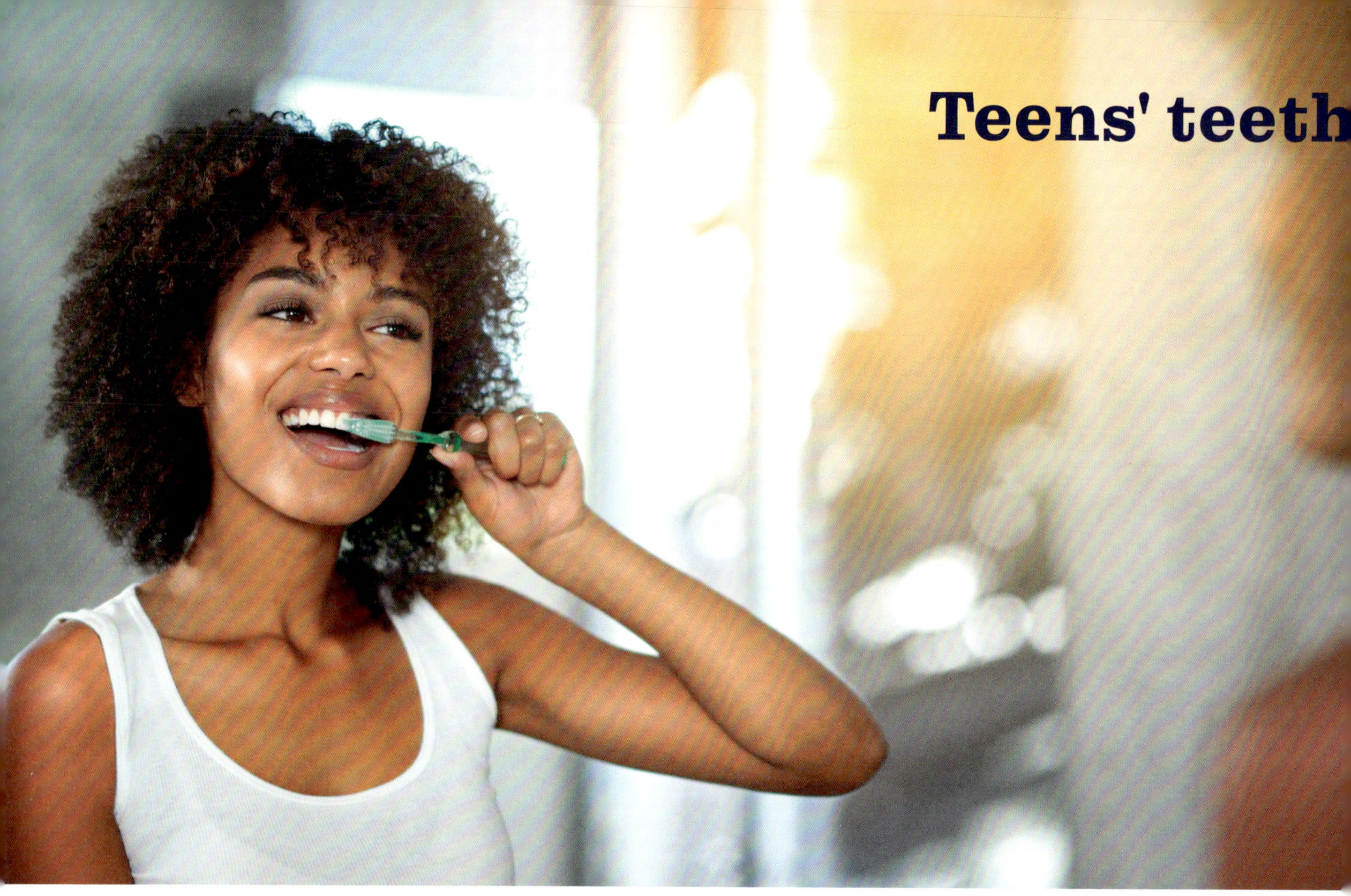

Why is a healthy smile important?

An attractive and healthy smile is important when meeting people and making friends. And it can boost your confidence and help you feel good about yourself.

If you don't look after your teeth and gums properly you could suffer from a number of different conditions that will make you stand out from the crowd for all the wrong reasons:

- Bad breath
- Stained teeth
- Tooth decay
- Gum disease
- Tooth loss
- Dental erosion.

Why is a healthy diet important for my oral health?

Every time you eat or drink anything sugary, your teeth are under acid attack for up to one hour. This is because the sugar reacts with the bacteria in plaque and produces harmful acids. Plaque is a build-up of bacteria which forms on your teeth.

It is better to have three or four meals a day rather than lots of snacks.

What is dental erosion?

Dental erosion is the gradual loss of tooth enamel caused by acid attacks. Enamel is the hard, protective coating of the tooth. If it is worn away, the dentine underneath is exposed and your teeth can look discoloured and become sensitive.

Drink up

Acidic foods and drinks and fizzy drinks cause dental erosion

Still water and milk are the best things to drink. Tea without sugar is also good for teeth as it contains fluoride.

Drink fruit juice just at mealtimes. If you want to drink fruit juices between meals, try diluting them with water.

Snacks

Avoid sugary snacks. If you need to eat between meals try these foods instead:

- Plain popcorn
- Nuts
- Cheese
- Breadsticks
- Plain yogurt
- Rice cakes
- Unsweetened cereal
- Plain bagels
- Fresh soup
- Raw vegetable pieces
- Fresh fruit.

What effects will smoking, alcohol or taking drugs have on my oral health?

Smoking can cause tooth staining, gum disease, tooth loss and – more seriously – mouth cancer. Smoking is also one of the main causes of bad breath.

Alcoholic drinks can also cause mouth cancer. If you smoke and drink you are more at risk.

Alcohol can also increase the risk of tooth decay and erosion. Some alcoholic drinks have a lot of sugar in them, and some mixed drinks may contain acids. So they can cause decay or dental erosion if you drink them often and in large amounts.

Illegal drugs can lead to a range of health problems. Smoking cannabis can have the same effects as smoking tobacco. Other drugs can cause a dry mouth and increase the risk of erosion, decay, gum disease and bad breath. Drugs can also cause you to grind your teeth, which can cause headaches and other problems. Many drugs can cause a craving for sugar, such as sweets and fizzy drinks, which can case tooth decay.

The human papillomavirus (HPV) is the main cause of cervical cancer and affects the skin that lines the moist areas of the body (such as the mouth). It can be spread through oral sex. Practising safe sex and limiting the number of partners you have may help reduce your chances of getting HPV.

You may hear about teenage girls and boys being offered the HPV vaccine to help prevent the virus. Talk to someone at your medical practice, or your parents or guardians, if you want to know more about this.

Your dentist may ask you questions about your lifestyle choices and general health because these may affect the health of your mouth.

How do I look?

Some people are unhappy with how their teeth look and feel self-conscious smiling in photos or in social situations. But you can have treatment to correct any problems.

How can I improve my smile?

An orthodontic appliance ('brace') will straighten or move your teeth to improve their appearance and the way they work. It can also help to improve the long-term health of your teeth, gums and jaw joints by spreading the biting pressure over all the teeth.

There are many different types of brace and your dental team or orthodontist will be able to talk to you about what is best for you.

Many people want to have whiter teeth. The only person who can whiten your teeth legally for you is a dentist, although there are 'home whitening kits' you can buy, you need to be over 18 to purchase these.

How long will I need to wear a brace?

It depends on how severe the problem is, and it may take anything from a few months to two-and-a-half years. However, most people can be treated in one to two years.

What is tooth jewellery?

Tooth jewellery involves sticking small jewels onto the teeth using dental cement. They should be fitted by a dentist, who can also easily remove them if necessary.

It is important to keep the area around the jewel clean, as plaque can easily build up around it and you will be more likely to get tooth decay.

What are the dangers of mouth piercing?

- Infection
- The surrounding tissues can become inflamed
- Blood infections
- The tongue can swell
- Teeth can chip and break
- It can be difficult to talk, eat and swallow
- It is difficult to keep your mouth clean
- Dental treatment can be difficult.

How can I protect my teeth when playing sports?

A mouthguard will help protect you against broken and damaged teeth, and even a broken or dislocated jaw.

It is important to wear a professionally made mouthguard whenever you play any sport that involves contact or moving objects.

Ask your dental team about a mouthguard. It is a small price to pay for peace of mind.

Top tips for teens

- Brush your teeth last thing at night and at least one other time during the day. Use a toothbrush with a small- to medium-sized brush head with soft to medium bristles, and brush for two minutes.
- You should use a pea-sized amount of toothpaste that contains 1,350ppm to 1,500ppm fluoride.
- Have sugary food and drinks just at mealtimes.
- Visit your dental team at least once a year, or as often as they recommend.
- Clean in between your teeth with 'interdental' brushes or floss at least once a day, to help remove plaque and food from between your teeth.
- Use a mouthwash to freshen your breath and kill bacteria.
- Use a straw if you have fizzy drinks, as this helps the drink to go to the back of your mouth and reduces the number of acid attacks on your teeth.
- Wait for at least one hour after eating or drinking anything acidic before you brush your teeth.
- Chew sugar-free gum after eating to help make more saliva and cancel out the acids which form in your mouth after eating.

The above information is reprinted with kind permission from Oral Health Foundation.

www.dentalhealth.org

How to keep your teeth clean

Brush your teeth with fluoride toothpaste twice a day for about 2 minutes to help keep you teeth and mouth healthy.

Plaque is a film of bacteria that coats your teeth if you don't brush them properly. It contributes to gum disease and tooth decay.

Tooth brushing stops plaque building up. Try to make sure you clean every surface of all your teeth.

When should I brush my teeth?

Brush your teeth for about 2 minutes last thing before you go to bed and on one other occasion every day.

Your dentist or hygienist may give you more advice based on your own dental health and needs.

Should I use an electric or manual toothbrush?

It doesn't matter whether you use an electric or manual toothbrush.

They're both equally good, as long as you clean all the surfaces of all your teeth and you use fluoride toothpaste.

But some people find it easier to clean their teeth thoroughly with an electric toothbrush.

What should I look for in a toothbrush?

For most adults, a toothbrush with a small head and compact, angled arrangement of long and short round end bristles is fine. Medium or soft bristles are best for mos people.

If you're using an electric brush, one with an oscillating o rotating head may work better than a manual toothbrush.

But making sure you thoroughly clean your teeth at leas twice a day is more important than the type of brush yo use. If in doubt, ask your dentist.

What type of toothpaste should I use?

It's important to use a toothpaste with the right concentratio of fluoride.

Check the packaging to find out how much fluoride each brand contains.

- Adults should use a toothpaste that contains at leas 1,350 parts per million (ppm) fluoride.
- Children don't need to use special children's toothpaste Children of all ages can use family toothpaste, as long a

How to brush your teeth

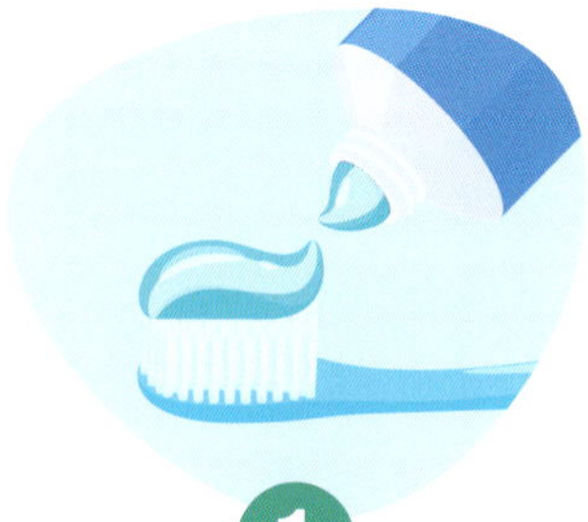

1

Apply toothpaste on a toothbrush

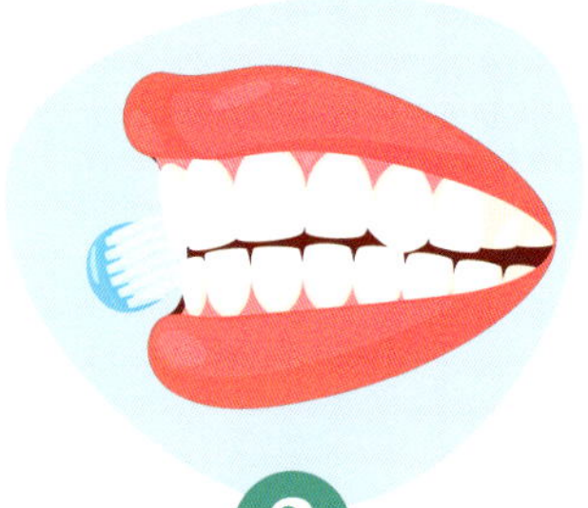

2

Place your brush at a 45 degree angle against your gum line.

Gently start to brush your teeth in short circular strokes away from the gum line.

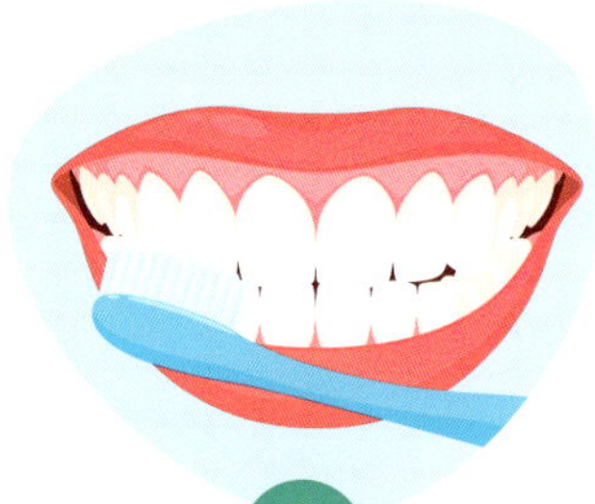

3

Using short back and forth strokes, gently brush all the surfaces in your mouth.

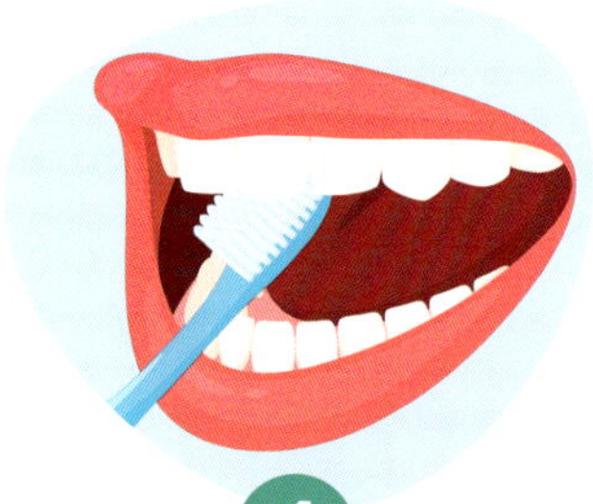

4

Clean the inner surfaces of your top teeth

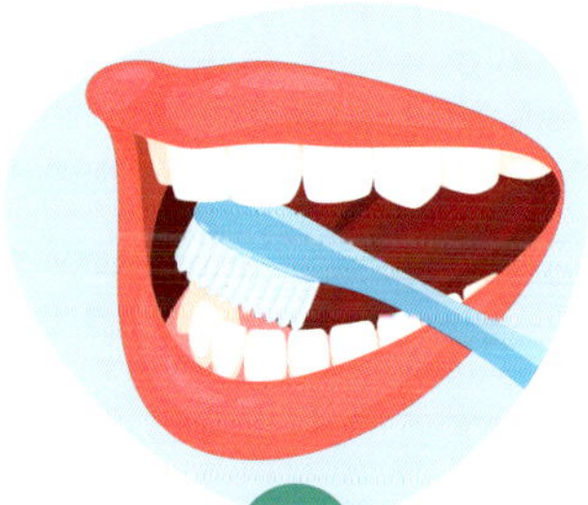

5

Clean the inner surfaces of your bottom teeth

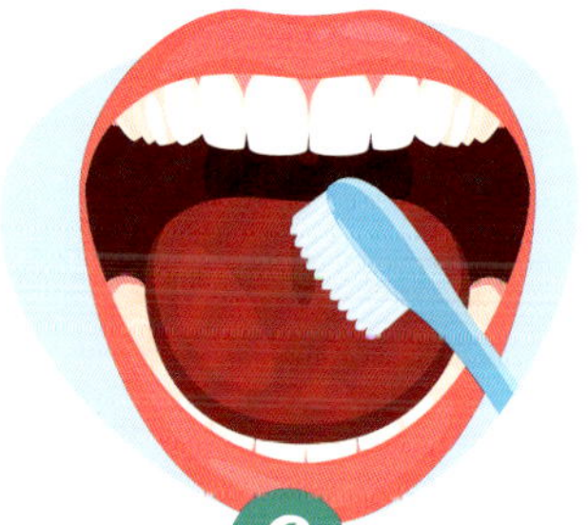

6

Clean your tongue

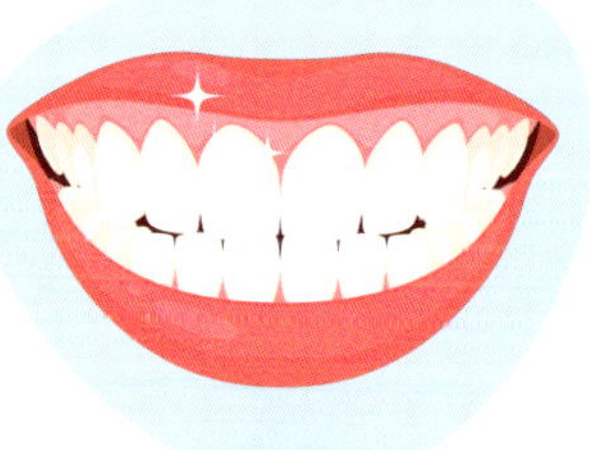

7

Done! Your smile is brilliant!

Rinsing
- Spit out toothpaste after brushing.
- Don't rinse with water – it washes away the fluoride that protects your teeth.

Mouthwash
- Don't use it straight after brushing. Best to use it later (like after lunch).
- Don't eat or drink for 30 mins after.
- Pick alcohol-free mouthwash.

Flossing
- Floss before brushing to get food out.

Interdental Brushes
- Clean between teeth to stop gum disease and bad breath.
- Good if you have bigger gaps.
- Never use toothpicks – they damage gums.

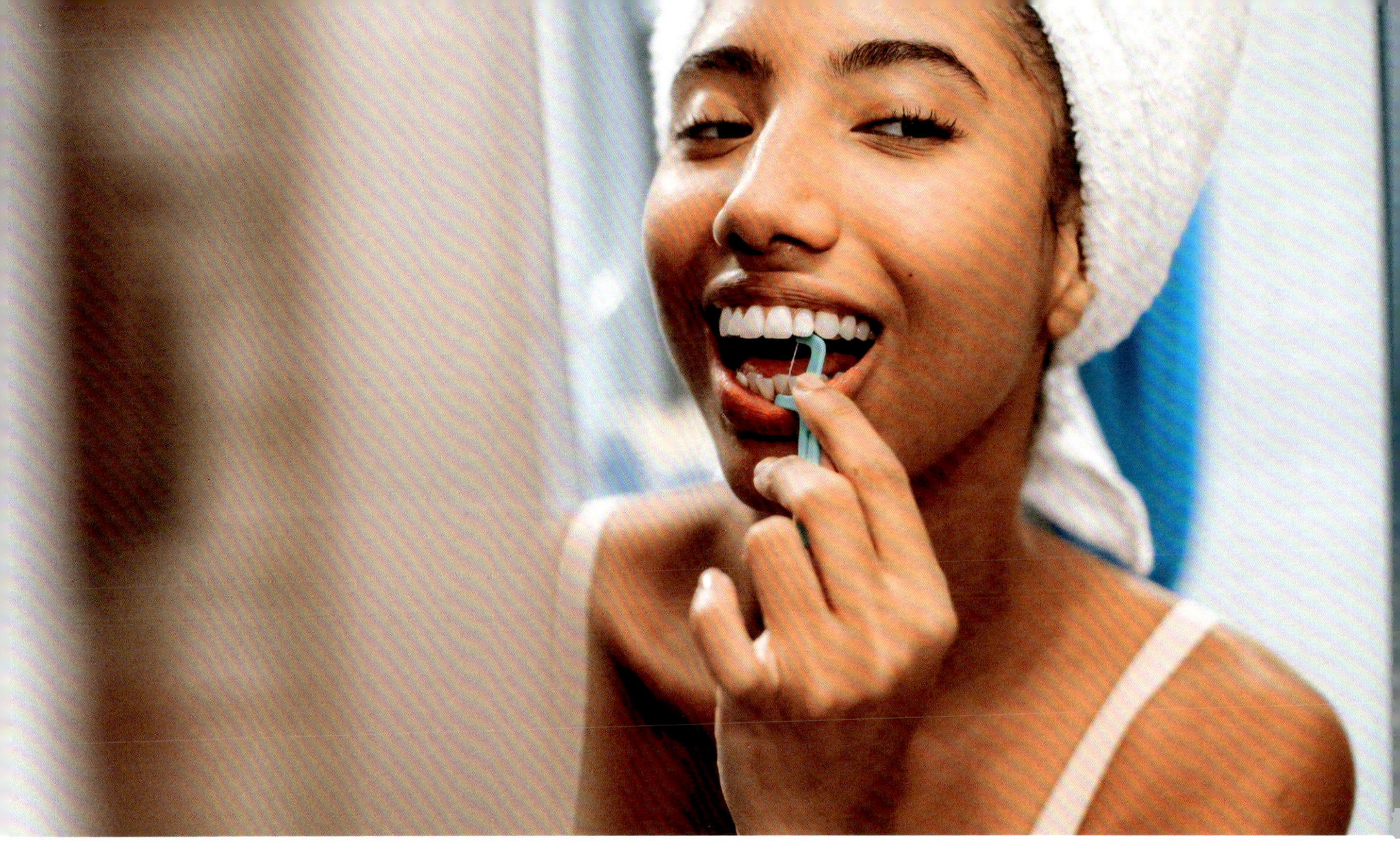

it contains 1,350 to 1,500ppm fluoride. Children aged 3 and under who don't have tooth decay can use a lower strength children's toothpaste, but make sure it contains at least 1,000ppm fluoride.

Children under the age of 3 should use just a smear of toothpaste. Children aged 3 to 6 years should use a pea-sized blob of toothpaste. Make sure children don't lick or eat toothpaste from the tube.

'our dentist may advise you or your child to use a toothpaste vith a higher concentration of fluoride, if you need it.

How to brush your teeth

Aake sure you clean all the surfaces of all your teeth, which hould take about 2 minutes.

emember to brush the inside surfaces, outside surfaces nd the chewing surfaces of your teeth.

Don't rinse with water straight after toothbrushing

fter brushing, spit out any excess toothpaste.

on't rinse your mouth immediately after brushing, as 'll wash away the concentrated fluoride in the remaining oothpaste.

insing dilutes it and reduces its preventative effects.

Should I use mouthwash?

sing a mouthwash that contains fluoride can help prevent ooth decay, but don't use mouthwash (even a fluoride one) traight after brushing your teeth or it'll wash away the oncentrated fluoride in the toothpaste left on your teeth.

hoose a different time to use mouthwash, such as after unch.

on't eat or drink for 30 minutes after using a fluoride nouthwash.

How to use dental floss

Flossing isn't just for dislodging food wedged between your teeth.

Regular flossing may also reduce gum disease and bad breath by removing plaque that forms along the gum line.

It's best to floss before brushing your teeth.

Take 30cm to 45cm of floss or dental tape and grasp it so you have 3cm or 4cm of floss taut between your hands.

Slip the floss or dental tape between the teeth and into the area between your teeth and gums, as far as it'll go.

Floss with 8 to 10 strokes, up and down between each tooth, to dislodge food and plaque.

How to use interdental brushes

You can use interdental brushes or single-tufted brushes instead of flossing, especially if there are gaps between your teeth.

The brush should fit snugly between the teeth.

Never use toothpicks to remove trapped food from between your teeth as you may damage your gums, which could lead to an infection.

Your dentist or hygienist can advise you on the best way to clean between your teeth.

15 February 2022

The experts: dentists on 22 quick, easy ways to care for your teeth

When's the best time to use mouthwash? Are interdental brushes better than floss? And shoulc you scrape your tongue? Here's the full lowdown on how to avoid decay and protect your gums

By Sarah Phillips

It's easy to take our dental health for granted until there is a problem – and then it can be a nightmare even getting an appointment. But most people have some level of gum disease, and even if it doesn't hurt, it may lead to worse problems further down the line. Here is advice from dentists on how to avoid painful and costly treatment.

Remember that sugar really is bad for your teeth

'We can't avoid sugar in modern diets – it is hidden everywhere,' says Tristan Roberts, a dentist who works at several private clinics in central London. 'The only reason we have tooth decay is because of sugar.' It is striking, says Roberts, that when we look at teeth in prehistoric skulls, there is hardly any sign of decay – and yet there weren't dentists and fillings back then. 'As soon as we started introducing refined sugars into the diet, decay exploded. Sugar itself doesn't cause decay but it causes bacteria in the mouth to go crazy: they eat the sugar and release lots of acid.'

Don't forget your (electric) toothbrush

'If you are going to have sugar, make sure you are brushing your teeth really well,' says Roberts. 'In this day and age, everybody should have an electric toothbrush. It doesn't have to be a top-of-the-range one, just rechargeable, as they work better, and ideally with a pressure sensor to make sure you're brushing gently around each tooth. And then it is a case of thoroughly brushing. You need to do the front, middle, back and sides of all your teeth, especially over the gum line, so you're not just brushing over the tops of them quickly.'

Cut down on snacks

'The timing of when we have sugar is just as important as the amount,' says Roberts. Limit eating and drinking sweet things to no more than four times a day: breakfast, lunch, dinner and one snack, he says. If you have to have chocolate, make sure it is at those times, 'rather than constantly grazing throughout the day when your teeth would be in a constant state of attack'. Rinsing your mouth out with water or using sugar-free chewing gum straight after a sugar hit can help to reduce the acidic load on the teeth, he says.

'Your teeth can cope with breakfast, lunch and tea, but they can't really cope with much else in between, other than water,' says NHS dentist Jenna Murgatroyd, who owns St Agnes Dental Practice in Cornwall. 'If you are constantly bathing your teeth in food, then you are constantly feeding the bacteria, which causes decay.'

Wait for 30 minutes after eating to brush

The saliva in our mouths is really good stuff for cleaning says Roberts. 'It has got things in it such as calcium and phosphate, which is what teeth are made of, causing th teeth to go into a state of repair.' It takes about half an hou after eating for saliva to remineralise the teeth, he says, s hold off on brushing until this point or you may end u brushing away the surface of your teeth. 'Your teeth hav the ability to reharden after you've eaten something,' say Murgatroyd. 'If you're brushing your teeth as soon as you'v eaten, then you are brushing off the softened enamel befor it has the chance to toughen up again.'

Brush before breakfast and last thing at night...

You don't need to brush your teeth every time you ea says Roberts – twice a day will suffice. 'Ideally, first thing i the morning to get the fluoride benefit of the toothpast protecting teeth during the day, and then especially we last thing at night, because when we sleep our mouths ar a lot drier; we haven't got the same amount of saliva that i produced during the day. Bacteria love those conditions an are a lot more likely to cause issues.'

...and keep at it for the full two minutes

'Most people will brush for less than a minute and think has been two minutes,' says Dr Praveen Sharma, an associat professor and honorary consultant in restorative dentistr at the Birmingham dental hospital and a scientific adviser t the British Dental Association. 'Even people with an electri toothbrush often don't realise that most have an inbui timer, which buzzes at certain intervals and buzzes a b differently when the full two minutes is up.'

Use fluoride toothpaste

'Fluoride makes the teeth about 10 times more resistant t erosion and decay,' says Roberts. 'It also has antibacteria properties that help to protect the teeth.'

Are fears about fluoride unfounded? Most areas in th UK don't have fluoridated water. In some places it occur naturally, and some councils add fluoride to the water suppl but in minute concentrations (one part of fluoride per millio parts of water). 'You're not going to get a significant amoun of fluoride exposure if you are brushing your teeth twice day, even if you're using high-strength fluoride toothpast Roberts explains. 'Yes, it can be dangerous if you're havin loads – say 1,000 times more fluoride than you would inges from brushing your teeth. And too much fluoride can weake

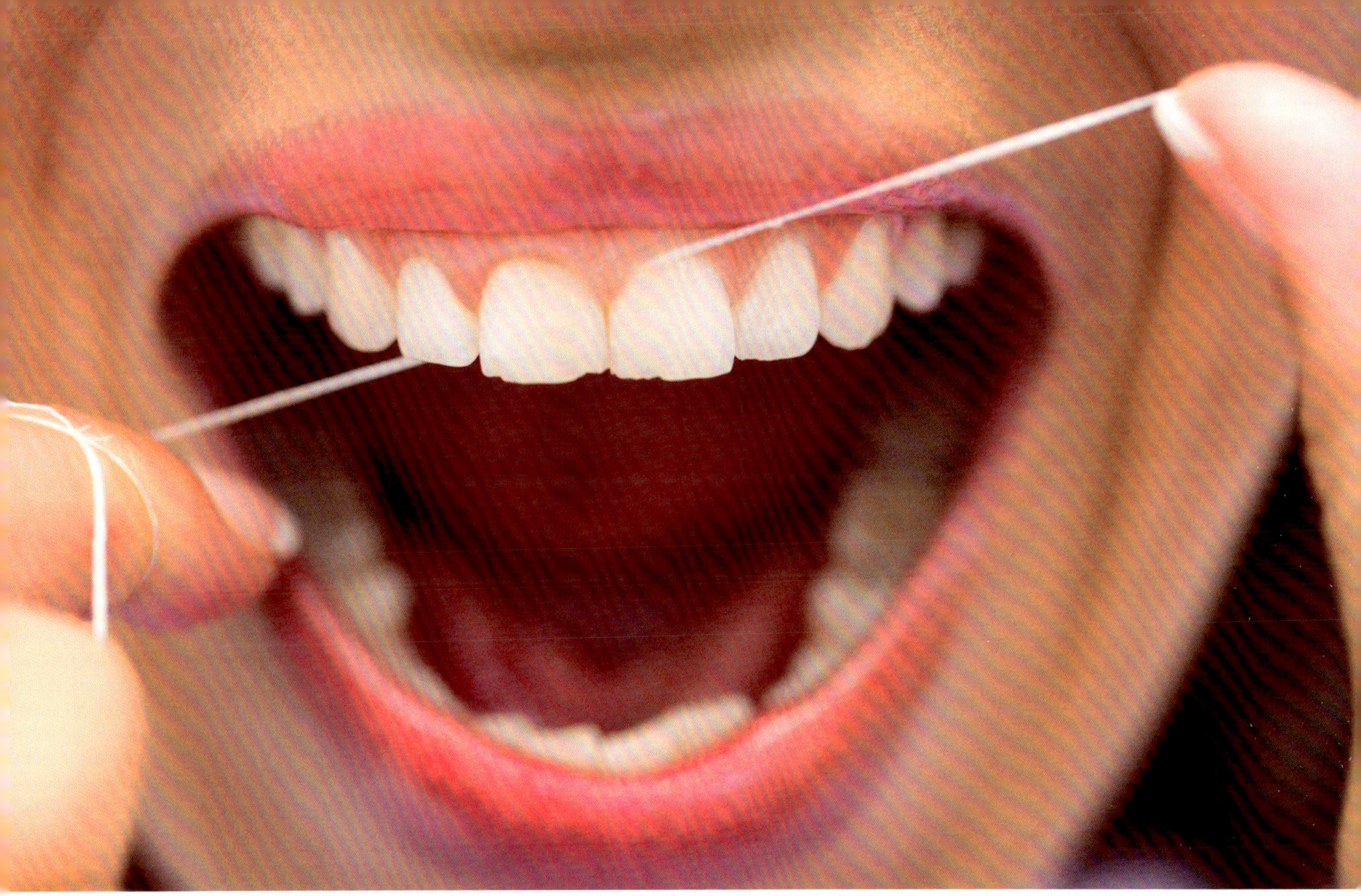

our teeth. So it's just about the sweet spot of having a little it of fluoride; you'll be fine with the concentrations that we ave available.' A smear of toothpaste for kids under three nd a tiny pea-size blob on a brush for kids aged three to six plenty, Roberts says.

Don't rinse

Spit the toothpaste out but don't rinse it with anything fterwards,' says Murgatroyd, to ensure you get the benefit om the toothpaste.

Avoid using mouthwash straight after brushing

t the moment, the advice is not to use mouthwash irectly after brushing your teeth,' says Roberts, 'because ne concentration of fluoride is a lot lower than what is in oothpaste. So either use it before brushing your teeth or ny other time during the day, half an hour after brushing.'

Brush mindfully

Brushing should be an exercise in mindfulness,' says Sharma, vhere you're really feeling the bristles going between the ooth and gums and from tooth to tooth, listening to the ound of the brush, tasting the toothpaste.' It should not be one 'while you're walking around doing other things at the ame time: you need to be very present in the moment'.

Don't forget to do both sides ...

f you're right-handed,' says Sharma, 'you tend to spend a lot nore time brushing the left side of the mouth instinctively, ecause it's easier to do, and you often neglect the right side. he reverse is true for left-handed people. When we're doing dental examination, we can guess whether someone's ght-handed or left-handed, because there's that level of difference in inflammation. For my right-handed patients, I advise them to start on the right and then work their way to the left. And vice versa for those who are left-handed.'

... and the rest of your mouth

'Although it's not essential for dental health, brushing your tongue daily will help prevent bad breath and reduce the number of potentially harmful microbes in the mouth,' says Roberts. Tongue scrapers are very useful tools for this, or a soft toothbrush can also be used.

You need to brush the gums as well, says Sharma: 'Angle the bristles down at 45 degrees for the bottom teeth and up at 45 degrees for the top teeth, so you are just sweeping below the gum line between the tooth and the gum, because that is an area that is often missed and where bacteria accumulates.' One of Sharma's specialisms is gum disease: 'Almost 90% of the population will have some level of gingivitis. You will notice redness, swelling or bleeding of the gums. Gingivitis is reversible by improving your brushing technique and visiting your dentist and hygienist.'

The more advanced form of gum disease is periodontitis, where the gum shrinks and teeth can eventually fall out. 'It's a real shame that periodontitis isn't a painful condition,' says Sharma, 'as it often goes unnoticed for decades.'

Don't wet your toothbrush

'We don't advise you to wet your toothbrush at all,' says Ajit Tanday, a fellow associate professor and consultant at Birmingham (Tanday and Sharma are married), who specialises in paediatric dentistry. 'Adding water to your toothbrush dilutes the toothpaste and encourages more foaming, so you spit out more of the toothpaste, as opposed to letting it sit on your teeth. This goes for everyone, not just children.'

Establish good routines as early as possible

'Children learn by mirroring,' says Tanday, 'so if you brush your teeth together as a family, they are probably going to be more inclined to do it because it's part of their routine.' She recommends gently rubbing a baby's gums with a muslin even before teeth erupt to establish the habit of cleaning. With young children, use an egg timer or app to ensure they brush for two minutes and help them to make sure a thorough job has been done. Tanday says she is often asked when a child can brush independently: it is something of a myth that if they can tie their shoelaces they can brush their teeth without help. 'My advice is to check every so often what their technique is like,' she says. The official guidance is until seven, but you definitely should keep an eye beyond this age, Tanday says.

Check up on the kids

Perhaps it's the result of having parents who are dentists, but Tanday has noticed that her child often fibs about brushing their teeth: 'They aren't a very good liar because the toothbrush is dry.' At weekends she gets around this by using a disclosing tablet after toothbrushing together: when chewed, the tablet temporarily stains plaque a bright colour, making it easy to spot the areas that need more attention.

Flossing is non-negotiable

'Interdental brushes – little brushes that go between the teeth – are the gold standard,' says Roberts. 'If you can't use them, standard floss is also good but it is technique-sensitive and we tend to do a better job with interdental brushes. Water flossers are better than nothing, but there's only so much plaque that can be removed by rinsing alone; the teeth need to be scrubbed in between.' If flossing makes your gums bleed, 'it is not from overbrushing, as some people think. They bleed because they have got inflammation. It just shows you need to clean them more frequently. The bleeding will stop after about a week if you are cleaning in between your teeth and brushing along the gums consistently.'

Manage stress

'Stress has a direct impact on your gum health by affecting your immune response,' says Sharma. 'You may already realise the impact of stress on your immune health if you've noticed that when you're stressed, you are more prone to get unwell. As periodontitis is an interplay between the bacteria in your mouth and your immune response to these bacteria, things that affect your immune response, such as stress, will affect your susceptibility to periodontitis.' There is also an indirect effect of stress because 'when you're stressed, you may neglect your oral hygiene. All of a sudden it is less of a priority to brush as well as you need to.'

Get tech on your side

Tanday suggests using an app, such as NHS food scanner, so you can see the sugar content of different foods compared with how much children should have a day. This can hel in developing an awareness of things such as cereal, whic is a big offender for hidden sugars. 'It's not about denyin children treats, but making swaps such as a square c chocolate instead of Haribo. Or giving them breadsticks an hummus as a snack rather than raisins, to reduce the suga intake even more.' Fruit is OK in moderation, although it acidity can be problematic, she says. Tanday reiterates th importance of limiting sugar to mealtimes rather than fo snacking.

Don't resort to DIY dentistry

'Most dental ailments are preventable with good ora hygiene at home and a good diet,' says Murgatroyd. 'I don recommend DIY dentistry, because you can do quite a lo of damage trying to pull out your own teeth and there ca be complications, too. Try to get an emergency dentis appointment as soon as possible.'

Try not to be scared of going to the dentist

'We understand that we're not everybody's favourite plac to visit,' says Murgatroyd. 'We are trained in looking afte people who are nervous about coming to see us, but th sooner you can pluck up the courage to come in, the soone we'll be able to look after you and help guide you wit your oral health journey.' That said, it is quite hard to acces dentistry on the NHS in the UK, she acknowledges. 'Th government is making it harder and harder for NHS practice to remain NHS, and that is a combination of funding and th contract itself. So it is very difficult to get an NHS dentist a the moment. On the NHS website, it is possible to searc practices to see if they might be taking on new patients. Bu generally practices don't have a waiting list for NHS patient

Having a filling is probably for the best

'We will never force you to have fillings,' says Murgatroyc 'but if we suggest them, it will be because you have decay i a tooth. If this decay is left, we may not be able to save th tooth. Generally, if a tooth is sore, the decay has gone to far and we need to either complete a root canal treatment, this is possible, or extract the tooth.'

A little of what you fancy does you good

Finally, remember that everything is OK in moderatior even dentists sometimes indulge. 'I would like to say on th record that I comply with all my instructions I give to m patients,' laughs Sharma. 'No – I have my vices, obviously. enjoy fizzy drinks and I have a sweet tooth. But then again, have excellent dental care available.'

31 October 2024

Is it better to shower in the morning or at night? Here's what a microbiologist say

An article from The Conversation.

By Primrose Freestone, Senior Lecturer in Clinical Microbiology, University of Leicester

It's a question that's long been the cause of debate: is it better to shower in the morning or at night?

Morning shower enthusiasts will say this is the obvious vinner, as it helps you wake up and start the day fresh. Night hower loyalists, on the other hand, will argue it's better to vash the day away' and relax before bed.

3ut what does the research actually say? As a microbiologist, can tell you there actually is a clear answer to this question.

irst off, it's important to stress that showering is an integral part of any good hygiene routine – regardless of when you orefer to have one.

howering helps us remove dirt and oil from our skin, which an help prevent skin rashes and infections.

howering also removes sweat, which can quell body odour.

lthough many of us think that body odour is caused by weat, it's actually produced by bacteria that live on the urface of our skin. Fresh sweat is, in fact, odourless. But kin-dwelling bacteria – specifically staphylococci – use weat as a direct nutrient source. When they break down he sweat, it releases a sulphur-containing compound called hioalcohols which is behind that pungent BO stench many f us are familiar with.

Day or night?

During the day, your body and hair inevitably collect pollutants and allergens (such as dust and pollen) alongside heir usual accumulation of sweat and sebaceous oil. While ome of these particles will be retained by your clothes, thers will inevitably be transferred to your sheets and illow cases.

he sweat and oil from your skin will also support the growth f the bacteria that comprise your skin microbiome. These acteria may then also be transferred from your body onto our sheets.

howering at night may remove some of the allergens, weat and oil picked up during the day so less ends up on our bedsheets.

owever, even if you've freshly showered before bed, you ill still sweat during the night – whatever the temperature . Your skin microbes will then eat the nutrients in that sweat. his means that by the morning, you'll have both deposited nicrobes onto your bed sheets and you'll probably also vake up with some BO.

Vhat particularly negates the cleaning benefits of a night hower is if your bedding is not regularly laundered. The odour causing microbes present in your bed sheets may be transferred while you sleep onto your clean body.

Showering at night also does not stop your skin cells being shed. This means they can potentially become the food source of house dust mites, whose waste can be allergenic. If you don't regularly wash your sheets, this could lead to a build-up of dead skin cell deposits which will feed more dust mites. The droppings from these dust mites can trigger allergies and exacerbate asthma.

Morning showers, on the other hand, can help remove dead skin cells as well as any sweat or bacteria you've picked up from your bed sheets during the night. This is especially important to do if your sheets weren't freshly washed when you went to bed.

A morning shower suggests your body will be cleaner of night-acquired skin microbes when putting on fresh clothes. You'll also start the day with less sweat for odour-producing bacteria to feed on – which will probably help you smell fresher for longer during the day compared to someone who showered at night. As a microbiologist, I am a day shower advocate.

Of course, everyone has their own shower preference. Whatever time you choose, remember that the effectiveness of your shower is influenced by many aspects of your personal hygiene regime – such as how frequently you wash your bed sheets.

So regardless of whether your prefer a morning or evening shower, it's important to clean your bed linen regularly. You should launder your sheets and pillow cases at least weekly to remove all the sweat, bacteria, dead skin cells and sebaceous oils that have built up on your sheets.

Washing will also remove any fungal spores that might be growing on the bed linen – alongside the nutrient sources these odour producing microbes use to grow.

19 May 2025

Is it true that ... showering every day is bad for your skin?

Does the length of time you stand in the water make a difference? And what about the temperature?

By Kate Lloyd

'If you'd asked me a couple of months ago, my answer might have been different,' says Dr Rosalind Simpson, a medical dermatologist at the University of Nottingham.

Historically, she says, daily washing was seen as problematic. It was thought that it might alter the skin's microbiome, stripping away natural protective oils and beneficial bacteria. People also worried that it might dry out the skin, causing cracks that allow bacteria and allergens to penetrate, potentially leading to infections and flare-ups of conditions such as eczema and psoriasis.

'But our department recently completed a randomised controlled trial on bathing in eczema patients, and the results are surprising,' she says.

The trial involved 438 eczema patients split into two groups: one that was asked to have a bath or shower six or more times a week; the other only once or twice weekly. 'You'd expect daily bathing to dry out the skin more and worsen eczema symptoms, but it didn't,' says Simpson. 'The study found no difference in symptoms between those who bathed daily and those who bathed less frequently.' Her takeaway? Frequency of washing doesn't correlate with increased skin dryness – and she believes this is true whether we have eczema or not.

The type of shower you take could increase irritation, though, Simpson adds. 'The longer you're in the water, the more it can dry out your skin, regardless of frequency. Shorter, cooler showers are better.' She says the shower gels, soaps and shaving products we choose can make a difference too. Ingredients such as methylisothiazolinone, methylchloroisothiazolinone, sulphates and parabens can cause reactions in some people. 'It's best to choose products with as few ingredients as possible, avoiding excessive fragrances and preservatives,' says Simpson. If you're experiencing irritation, she suggests using an emollient cream, instead of standard soap, to wash yourself.

Overall, she says, the best shower routine is the one that makes you feel good. 'Do what suits your skin – everyone's going to be different.'

31 March 2025

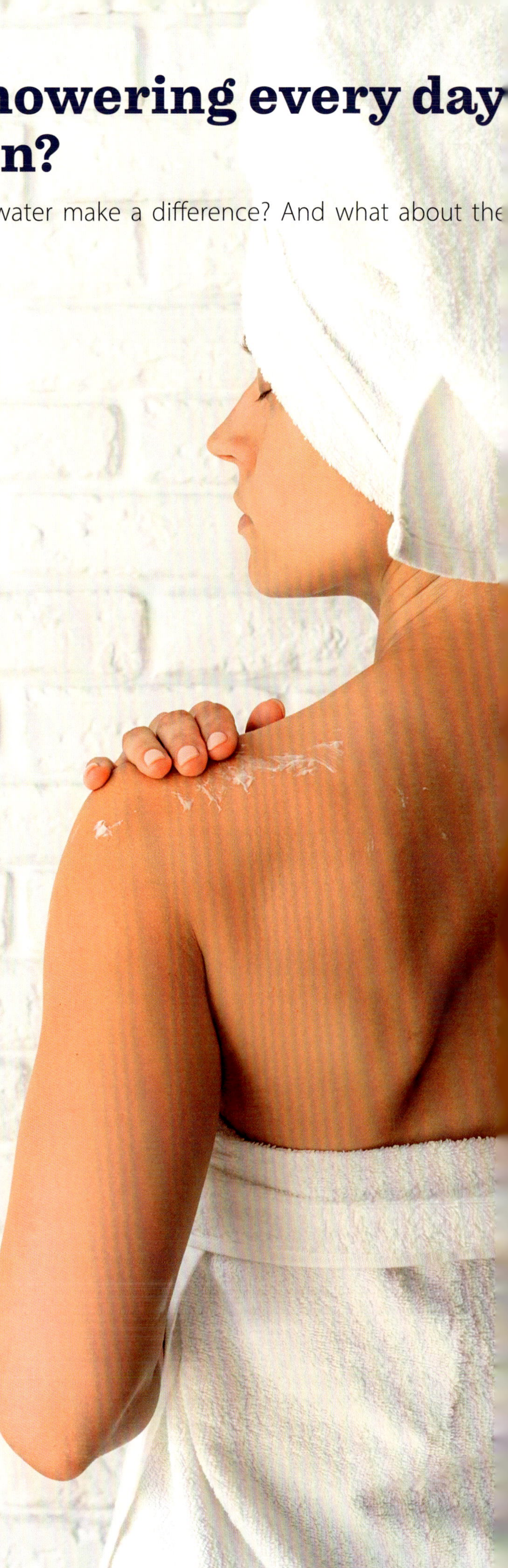

Why do I smell? Understanding body odour

Ever come home from school after PE or a hot day and thought, 'Wait… is that me?' Body odour (often called BO) is something most people worry about at some ›oint. It can feel embarrassing, but it's completely normal. 3O happens when sweat mixes with bacteria on your skin - it's not just about being 'dirty'. In this article we'll look at vhere BO shows up, what causes it, and how to deal with it.

Common areas for BO

›ome body parts are more likely to smell because they're varm, sweaty or don't get much air.

Armpits – lots of sweat glands make them one of the main sources of BO.

Groin area – heat and tight clothing mean sweat and odour can build up quickly.

Feet – trapped in socks and shoes, feet provide the perfect damp place for bacteria to grow.

Hair and scalp – natural oils and sweat can make hair greasy and smelly if it isn't washed.

Causes of BO

o why does BO actually happen? There are a few main easons:

Sweat – on its own, sweat doesn't smell. Odour starts when bacteria break it down.

Bacteria – harmless skin bacteria feed on sweat and release smelly chemicals.

Diet – foods like garlic, onions and spicy meals can affect how your body smells.

Hormones – puberty and periods make sweat glands more active, which is why teenagers often notice BO more.

Stress – stress sweat is thicker and produces a stronger odour.

How to treat and prevent BO

he good news? BO is totally manageable. Here are some ractical tips:

;ood hygiene

hower or bathe daily, especially after sport or exercise. Use n antibacterial soap or body wash and pay extra attention › armpits, groin and feet.

:lothing choices

lways put on clean clothes each day. Fabrics like cotton are reathable and help reduce sweating. Change socks and nderwear daily (or more often if you've been active).

Deodorants and antiperspirants

Deodorants mask odour, while antiperspirants reduce the amount you sweat. You can use either or both depending on what works for you. If you have sensitive skin, look for fragrance-free options.

Foot care

Wash your feet every day, dry them carefully (especially between the toes), and wear clean socks. Foot powders or sprays can help keep them dry and fresh. Let your shoes air out rather than wearing the same pair all the time.

Hair and scalp

Wash your hair regularly, particularly if you've been sweating. For people with longer hair, tying it up during sport can reduce sweat build-up on the scalp.

Diet and lifestyle

Drinking plenty of water helps your body flush out toxins. If you notice certain foods make your BO worse, try cutting down on them.

Managing stress

Relaxation techniques like deep breathing, exercise, or even talking things through with someone can lower stress – and reduce stress-related sweat.

When to see a doctor

If your body odour suddenly changes, gets stronger, or doesn't improve with good hygiene, it's worth checking in with your GP. Sometimes conditions like excessive sweating (hyperhidrosis) or infections need medical advice.

Fresh and confident

Body odour is a normal part of growing up, especially during puberty. Everyone sweats and everyone smells sometimes – but with the right habits, it doesn't have to be a big deal. Taking care of your hygiene not only keeps you smelling fresh but also boosts your confidence in school, with friends, and beyond.

Myth-busting quiz

Copy the following statements into your book and write true or false next to each one:

1. Sweat itself smells bad.
2. Eating lots of garlic can affect your body odour.
3. Stress can make your sweat smell stronger.
4. Wearing the same socks two days in a row has no effect on BO.
5. Everyone experiences body odour during puberty.

Whole-body deodorants: a solution to a non-existent problem

An article from The Conversation.

By Michelle Spear, Professor of Anatomy, University of Bristol

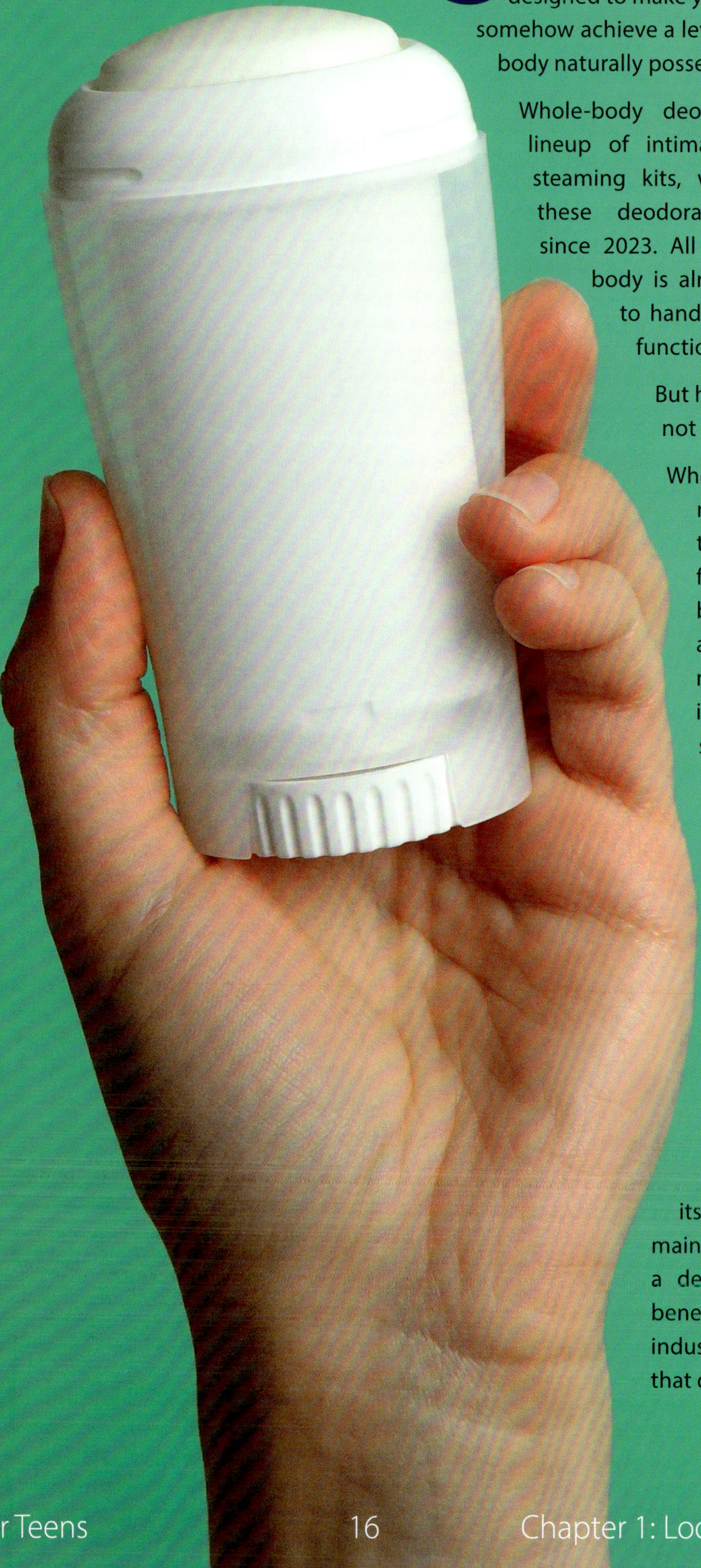

Step into any supermarket or pharmacy, anc you'll find aisles brimming with product designed to make you smell 'fresh', feel 'clean', o somehow achieve a level of 'purity' that no humar body naturally possesses.

Whole-body deodorants have joined the lineup of intimate washes, douches anc steaming kits, with internet searches fo these deodorants massively increasing since 2023. All promise to do what you body is already masterfully equippec to handle: keeping itself clean anc functioning.

But here's the thing, your body i not unclean.

Whole-body deodorants ar marketed for areas beyon the armpit, most commonl feet and intimate areas but the premise that thes areas are inherently dirty i misleading. In fact, the bod is a finely tuned biologica system that has been self regulating for millennia The notion that you nee expensive products t achieve basic hygien is a fallacy rooted i marketing, not science

Self-cleaning vaginas

The vagina is one of th most misunderstoo parts of the body when i comes to hygiene. Despit its remarkable ability t maintain its own health throug a delicate balance of pH an beneficial bacteria, an entir industry exists to sell product that disrupt this natural system.

rom douches to scented wipes, these products often cause he very issues they claim to solve, such as infections or rritation.

entral to the vagina's self-cleaning process is vaginal lischarge – a natural and essential function. Discharge onsists of water, mucus and cells shed from the vaginal ning, which flush out bacteria, dead cells and debris.

hanks to this continuous self-flushing mechanism, no nternal cleaning, such as douching, is necessary. In fact, uch interventions can disturb the vaginal microbiome, ncreasing the risk of bacterial vaginosis or yeast infections.

/aginal steaming, a practice promoted by wellness nfluencers, claims to 'cleanse' or 'revitalise' the uterus and agina. Yet there is no evidence of benefit and, in terms of the uterus, reveals a misunderstanding of anatomy. It is nnecessary at best and harmful at worst.

Vhile the vagina takes care of its internal health, the external ulval area does require some attention. Exposed to sweat, rine and natural oils, the vulval skin benefits from gentle laily cleaning with warm water or mild soap.

Male intimate hygiene

or men, the marketing approach differs but remains equally nisleading. Products like intimate washes and deodorising prays are presented as essential for modern grooming. onsider the rise of 'ball sprays' (a genuine term) and lotions, /hich promise to keep the scrotum dry and odour-free.

he scrotum is more than just a protective pouch for the estes; it is also a thermoregulating organ designed to naintain an optimal temperature for sperm production. To chieve this, the scrotum is equipped with eccrine sweat lands.

hese glands are small coiled structures located within the ermis of the skin. They function by releasing sweat through ucts that open directly onto the surface of the skin. This weat evaporates, dissipating heat and helping to cool the crotum.

nlike apocrine sweat glands found in areas such as the rmpits or groin, eccrine glands do not produce the lipid-ch secretions that can lead to body odour when broken own by bacteria, so scrotum sweat is typically odourless.

/hile excessive moisture can lead to issues such as fungal nfections, these are often managed with breathable fabrics, egular washing and thorough drying – not specialised roducts.

eet, often confined in socks and shoes, are another frequent arget of whole-body deodorants and sprays. Feet are not nherently dirty, they are simply hardworking, equipped with bout 250,000 sweat glands – the highest concentration of weat glands in the body.

Like the scrotum, these are eccrine sweat glands, releasing mostly water-based sweat to help cool the feet, particularly during physical activity or in warm conditions.

Moisture from sweat also reduces friction between the skin and footwear. Additionally, eccrine sweat keeps the skin of the feet supple and prevents cracking, which might otherwise create entry points for infections.

Though sweat from the feet is odourless when trapped in moist, warm environments such as socks or shoes, bacteria on the skin break down sweat components, releasing compounds that cause odour. Prolonged moisture can also lead to fungal infections, such as athlete's foot and skin maceration, where softened skin becomes more prone to irritation or breakdown.

Managing foot sweat involves supporting the body's natural processes rather than eliminating them. Daily washing with warm water and mild soap, followed by thorough drying, is essential.

So, the bottom line is, if a company is trying to sell you the idea that your body is inherently unclean, it's likely not your hygiene that needs fixing. It's their marketing pitch.

However, if body odour persists despite daily washing, it could signal an underlying medical condition. These conditions deserve sympathetic investigation and appropriate support, not masking with overpriced products that treat only the symptom rather than the cause.

23 January 2025

Spot the marketing tricks

Below are three examples of marketing tricks taken from the article. Copy them into your book and explain why each one is misleading.

1. Whole-body deodorants – marketed for areas beyond the armpits, like feet and intimate areas, suggesting those parts are dirty.
2. Douches, wipes, and steaming kits – sold as if the vagina needs extra cleaning, even though it naturally keeps itself healthy.
3. 'Ball sprays' and intimate washes for men – promoted as essential for grooming, even though scrotum sweat is usually odourless.

Hygiene tips

List five simple, low-cost ways to support your body's natural cleaning systems without buying unnecessary products.

How to clean your vagina

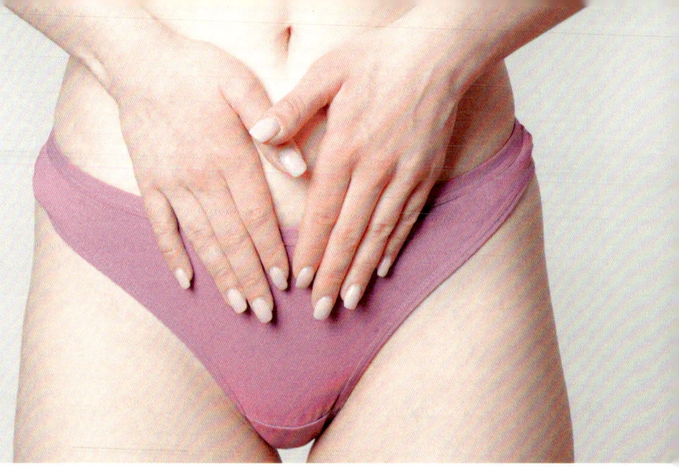

Many people are confused about whether they need to wash their vagina, and it is a question that comes up often. The short answer is: no, your vagina does not need cleaning because it cleans itself. What does need gentle washing is your vulva – the external part of your genitals. Understanding the difference between vagina and vulva is the first step to knowing how to look after your body in a healthy way.

What's the difference between vagina and vulva?

When most people say 'vagina', they often mean the whole area between their legs, but that is not quite right. Your vagina is actually an internal muscular tube. It runs from your cervix (the lower part of the womb) to the vaginal opening.

The external parts – the ones you can see – are called the vulva. This includes your vaginal opening, the lips (labia), your clitoris, the urethra (where urine leaves the body) and your pubic mound. Knowing the difference matters because the vagina looks after itself, while the vulva needs daily care.

How does the vagina clean itself?

Your vagina has its own built-in cleaning system. It produces natural secretions called vaginal discharge. This discharge contains healthy bacteria that keep the pH level balanced and help protect you from infections.

Because of this, you should not try to wash inside your vagina. Doing so can upset the balance of bacteria and actually cause more problems, not fewer. Discharge is completely normal, and it can change throughout your menstrual cycle. A mild smell is also normal – it is just your body doing its job.

The best way to wash your vulva

While your vagina takes care of itself, your vulva benefits from gentle daily washing. You might want to wash a little more often during your period, but you don't need to do anything complicated.

Here are some simple steps:

- Use warm water and, if you want, a mild unperfumed soap or a soap-free substitute.
- Wash with your hands rather than a sponge or cloth, which can be too rough.
- Be careful not to get soap inside your vagina.
- Wash the area between your vaginal opening and your anus (called the perineum).
- Always wash from front to back to avoid moving bacteria from your anus to your vulva.
- After washing, gently pat dry with a clean towel.

These steps are more than enough to keep your vulva healthy and clean.

Cleaning dos and don'ts

There are lots of products on the market that claim to make you 'fresh' or 'clean', but many of them are unnecessary and can even be harmful.

Do:

- ✓ Use plain soap or a soap substitute if you have sensitive skin.
- ✓ Use fragrance-free wipes only if you really need to freshen up, and make sure they are designed for the vulva.

Don't:

- ✗ Use perfumed washes, antiseptics or gels – these can upset the natural balance of bacteria.
- ✗ Try vaginal douching (flushing water up inside) – it removes the good bacteria you need to stay healthy.
- ✗ Experiment with vaginal steaming, which some celebrities promote. There is no scientific proof it helps and it can actually be dangerous.

Remember: your vagina is not supposed to smell like perfume. A light, natural smell is completely normal, and it can change during your cycle.

When to see a doctor

Sometimes your body will send you signals that something is not quite right. You should speak to a doctor or nurse if you notice:

- a strong or unpleasant smell
- unusual itching, soreness or irritation
- discharge that looks different from normal

These can all be signs of an infection. The good news is that most infections are common and easily treated, so there is no need to feel embarrassed about asking for help.

Freshness without the fuss

You do not need to clean your vagina – it has an amazing self-cleaning system. What you do need to do is gently wash your vulva every day with water and mild products. Keeping things simple is the healthiest choice.

'How do I clean my penis?'

An article by The Conversation.

By David King, Senior Lecturer in General Practice, The University of Queensland

> 'Growing up, no one ever gave me the rundown on how or what I should do to keep my penis clean [...] I've never read any reliable answer beyond washing it with water. Do I use soap? Any soap? How normal is smegma? If my penis gets itchy from smegma should I go see a doctor? If so, my GP or a urologist?' – Anonymous

Key points

- clean under the foreskin, using soap, but not too much
- smegma is normal
- if you have any concerns, see your GP.

It's a shame some people think talking about cleaning and caring for our genitals is embarrassing or taboo. We probably know more about hair care than penis care.

The penis is simply another part of our anatomy, so cleaning should be relatively straight forward.

If you've been circumcised, where your foreskin was removed soon after birth, your penis will look different, with the head (or glans) always exposed.

But if you have a foreskin, there are some extra things to think about when washing, which we'll get to soon.

Foreskin facts

But first, some foreskin facts. From around the time you turn five, your foreskin separates from the head of your penis, bit by bit. This allows you to pull back your foreskin (retract it). In some boys, the foreskin can stay partially stuck to the head of the penis until puberty.

You should never forcibly pull back your foreskin. That'll be painful, you could bleed, you could scar, or have other complications.

OK, now for the washing part

Once your foreskin separates easily from the glans, gently retract and clean underneath the foreskin with each bath or shower. Then, after washing, pull the foreskin forward to its normal position.

When it's time to dry off, retract the foreskin again so you can dry the head of the penis with a towel. Then, you guessed it, pull the foreskin forward to its normal position.

It's OK to clean with soap whether you have a foreskin or not. But generally, too much soap is worse than none at all. Excessive cleaning removes essential body oils that would normally keep our skin moist and reduce friction. If you have sensitive skin, you can use a soap-free wash from the chemist.

What about smegma?

Smegma is a thick, whitish discharge consisting of a build-up of dead skin cells, oil and other fluids under the foreskin. And it's very useful. It protects and lubricates the penis.

Some people have oilier skin than others and tend to have more smegma. So some smegma is normal, but if you have too much or it becomes smelly, you may need to clean more.

Things to watch out for (and when to see your GP)

If the head of your penis becomes painful, red, itchy and has a discharge, you may have a treatable condition called balanitis.

It's more common if you have a foreskin. And the bacteria and fungus that cause it like the warm and moist conditions under there.

Skin disorders, infection, poor hygiene, friction from sexual activity, and using too much soap all cause the condition.

You can clear a mild case with good hygiene and simple treatments, such as an antiseptic or antifungal cream. You can buy these from any pharmacy. In addition to the medication, the cream itself helps protect and moisturise the inflamed skin.

If you have balanitis you may need to be more careful than usual to avoid urine irritating your inflamed skin. Retract your foreskin when you urinate. Dry the head of the penis gently after you finish.

If your penis is still inflamed after a week of these simple measures it's best to see your GP. They can then investigate other causes, such as psoriasis or an allergy.

9 December 2019

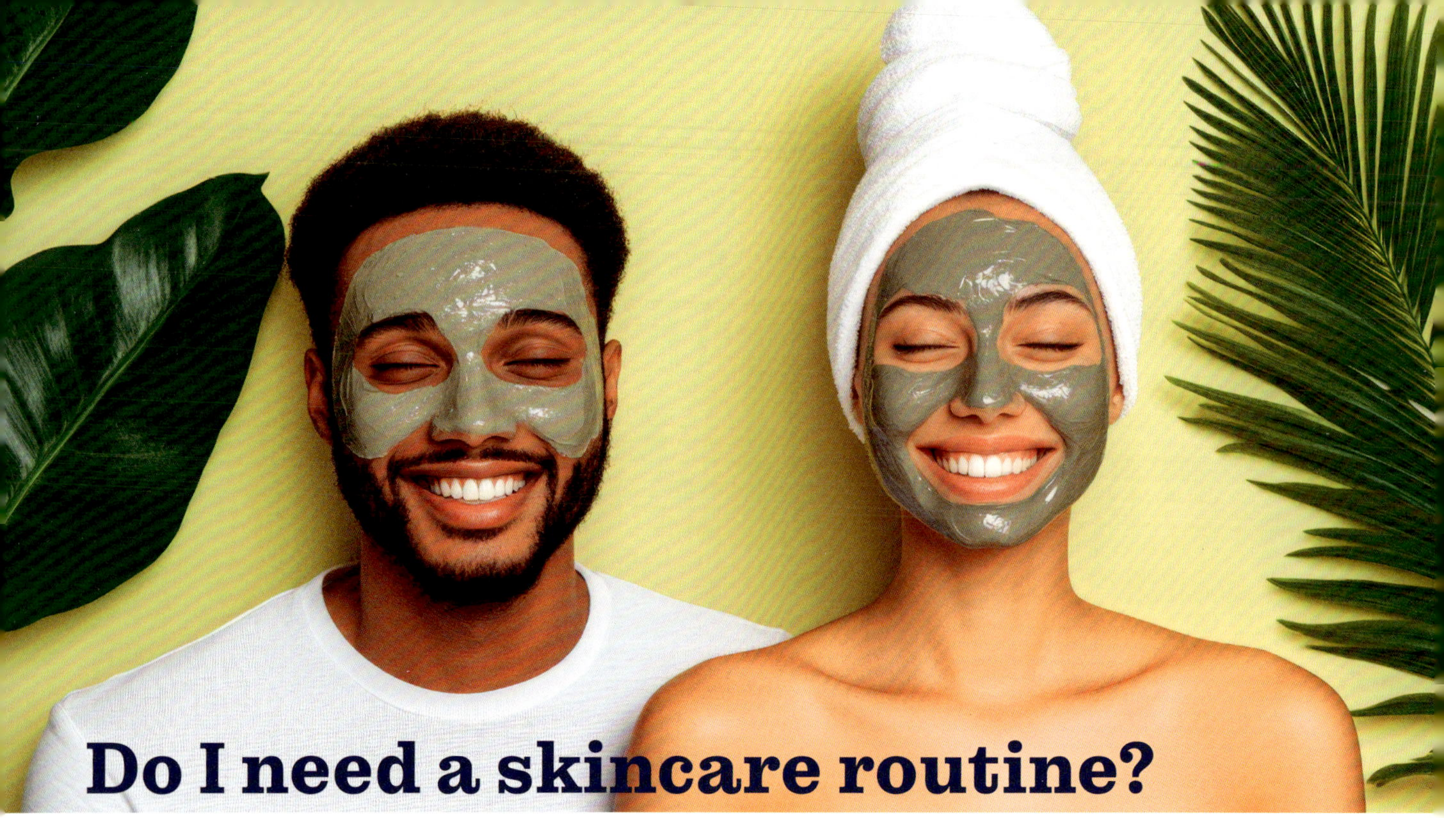

Do I need a skincare routine?

Walk into any shop or scroll through TikTok, and you'll quickly see rows of skincare products promising glowing, flawless skin. From fancy serums to 10-step routines, it can feel like everyone is doing something for their skin. But do you really need a complicated skincare routine? The short answer is no – healthy skin doesn't come from owning every product on the shelf.

What your skin really needs

Your skin is the largest organ in your body, and it's already very good at looking after itself. For most teenagers, the basics are enough: wash your face gently to remove sweat and dirt, use moisturiser if your skin feels dry or tight, and apply sunscreen during the day to protect from sun damage. That's it. A 'routine' doesn't need to be more complicated unless your skin has specific problems like acne or eczema. In fact, keeping things simple can prevent irritation and help your skin stay balanced.

The problem with overdoing it

It's tempting to believe that the more products you use, the better your skin will look. But piling on creams, serums, and acids can actually cause the opposite effect. Many products designed for adults contain strong active ingredients like retinol or chemical exfoliants. Teen skin is naturally more delicate and using these too early can lead to redness, burning, dryness, or even permanent sensitivity. If you've ever felt stinging after applying a product, that's your skin telling you it's too much. More does not always mean better – sometimes, less is healthier.

When a routine helps

That said, a simple routine can make a difference if you struggle with certain skin types. If your skin is oily or prone to breakouts, washing it gently twice a day and using an oil-free moisturiser may help. If your skin is very dry, a fragrance-free cream can soothe it. Sunscreen is always worth using because sun damage builds up over time, even when you're young. If spots or irritation don't improve with gentle care it's best to speak to your GP or a dermatologist instead of copying routines from TikTok. They can suggest treatments that actually work for teenage skin.

Myths about skincare

There are plenty of myths online about what you 'must' do for good skin. Here are a few worth busting:

- Myth 1: Everyone needs a 10-step skincare routine. Reality: You don't. The basics – cleansing, moisturising and protecting – are enough.
- Myth 2: Expensive products always work better. Reality: Simple, budget-friendly options can work just as well as luxury brands.
- Myth 3: More products clear spots faster. Reality: Overloading your skin can make acne worse and cause irritation.

Keep it simple

The truth is that your skin doesn't need dozens of products to be healthy. Drinking water, eating balanced meals, getting enough sleep, and managing stress are just as important as anything you put on your face. Skincare should feel easy, not overwhelming. If you stick to the basics and listen to what your skin is telling you, you'll already be doing enough.

Looking after your skin isn't about following trends – it's about keeping it healthy in a way that works for you.

Viral TikTok skincare routines can actually be harmful to teens, new study finds

;tudy found that skincare products contain ingredients that increase the risk of developing allergic contact dermatitis.

3y Amber Raiken

Viral skincare routines on TikTok could be doing more harm than good.

According to a new study published in the journal *'ediatrics* on Monday, two researchers at Northwestern Jniversity each created their own TikTok accounts and epresented themselves as 13-year-olds. They went on o discover relevant videos on their 'For You' pages on the pp, before compiling 100 unique clips of girls, aged 18 or 'ounger, sharing their skincare regimen.

After examining the footage from these content creators, the cientists gathered a list of products used in the videos. They vent on to identify products' active and inactive ingredients, n order to identify if they had an elevated risk of developing skin allergy known as allergic contact dermatitis.

Results of the study found that on average, girls between he ages of seven and 18 were using six different products on their faces, while others were using more than 12.

n the top-viewed TikTok videos included in the study, some of these products had an average of 11 potentially irritating ctive ingredients. As a result, researchers determined ontent creators were at risk of developing skin irritation, un sensitivity, and allergic contact dermatitis.

That high risk of irritation came from both using multiple ctive ingredients at the same time, such as hydroxy acids, s well as applying the same active ingredient unknowingly over and over again when that active ingredient was found in hree, four, five different products,' the study's corresponding uthor, Dr. Molly Hales, said in a press release.

One video specifically showed a girl applying 10 products on her face in six minutes.

As she's applying the products, she begins to express liscomfort and burning, and in the final few minutes, she levelops a visible skin reaction,' senior author of the study, Dr. Tara Lagu said.

'he study also found that these content creators pay a hefty rice for their skincare routines. In fact, each teenager's daily kincare routine costs an average of $168, with the study's uthors estimating that each product lasts at least a month, lepending on its size.

However, some skincare regimens demonstrated by teens on TikTok cost more than $500, depending on how many products they use every day.

The study about skincare came a year after tweens turned heads for taking over the aisles of Sephora. In late 2023, college student Chloe Grace took to TikTok to share her shopping experience at Sephora, and inadvertently sparked a viral phenomenon known as 'Sephora Kids.'

'Has anyone else noticed that every time you go into Sephora now, it's just all little girls?' she began the video.

TikTok user Megan Lacey also went viral when she detailed her Sephora encounter with a few tween girls 'taking up every single section' in the store. Just days later, TikTok user Dane recalled 'a group of three young girls' were 'rude' to him at a Sephora.

Social media is driving the 'Sephora kids' epidemic, with children as young as seven sharing their skincare routines on TikTok, Instagram, and YouTube. Children as young as 10 are also using anti-aging products, containing ingredients such as retinol, exfoliating acids, toners, and serums designed to minimise the effects of aging.

This has sparked heated debate, with some people claiming the clips are harmless fun. However, others, including dermatologists, have argued that young skin is too new and delicate for aggressive adult skincare products that could damage it and make it extra vulnerable to the sun.

9 June 2025

Think it through

Why do you think so many people your age feel pressured to have a complicated skincare routine? Write down two reasons and share with a partner.

True or false?

The basics of skincare are cleansing, moisturising, and sun protection. Do you agree? Explain your answer with one example.

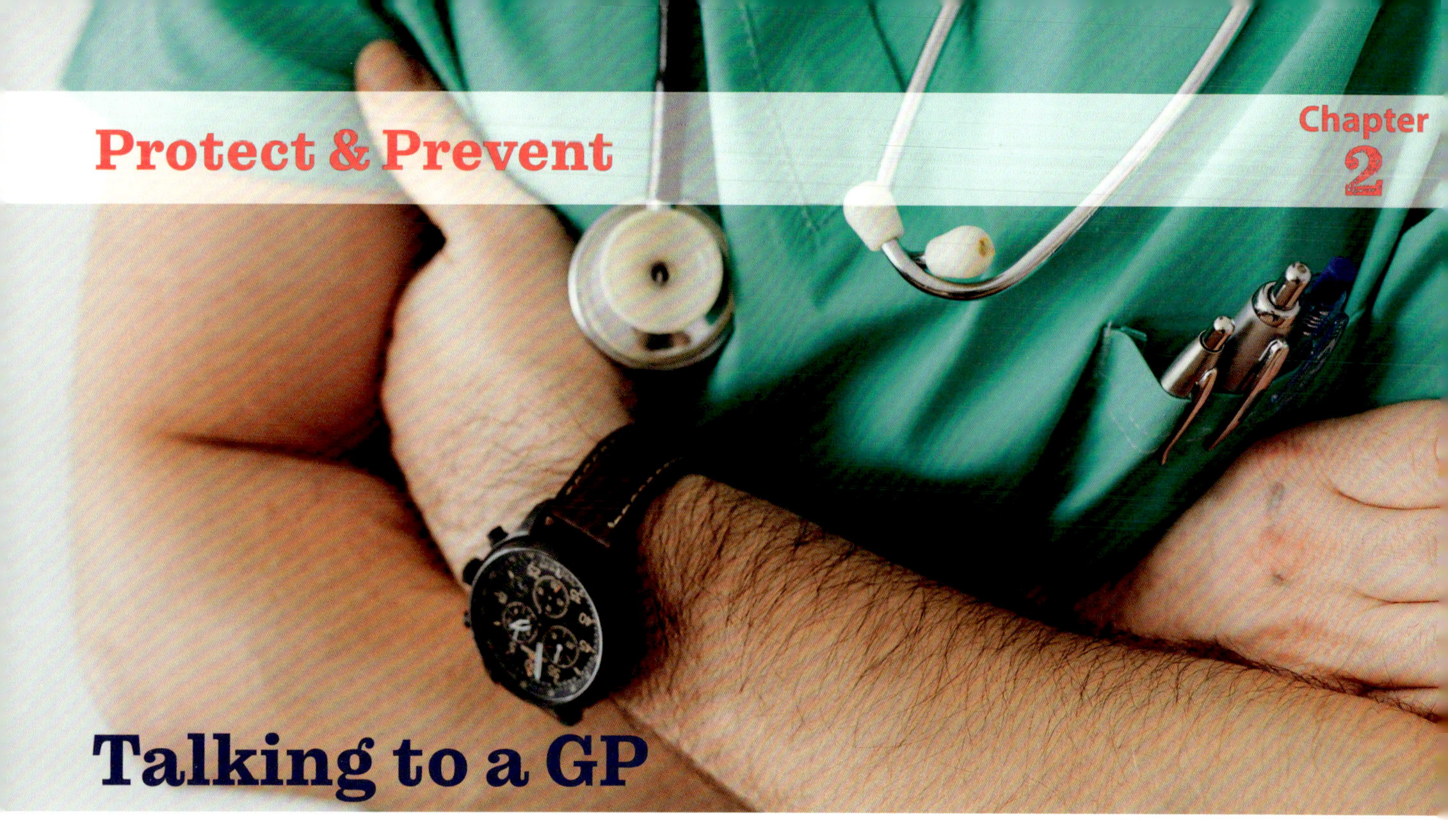

Talking to a GP

What is a GP?

A General Practitioner (GP) is a doctor who has extra training to work in the community, dealing with all kinds of health problems. You can speak to a GP about anything to do with your physical or mental health.

How to register at a GP surgery

If you're 16 or over, you can sign up to a GP surgery without the help of a parent or carer. If you're under 16, a parent or carer might need to fill out a registration form on your behalf.

Everyone has the right to register with a GP practice of their choice, and you don't have to sign up to the same GP practice as your family members if you don't want to.

However, a GP practice may be unable to register you if:

- They are not taking on new patients
- You do not live within its practice boundaries

To register, you might need to fill in a form and provide some proof of your identity and address, such as a passport and a letter addressed to you. GP surgeries can have different registration processes, so call them or visit their reception to find out what information they need from you.

Booking an appointment

You can book your own GP appointment at any age. All surgeries have different systems for booking appointments.

To book an appointment, you'll need to contact your GP surgery and arrange an appointment. You might be asked about the reason for your appointment, this is just to make sure you receive the right care. You don't have to tell them if you don't want to, just say it's personal.

You can also request to see a male or female GP if you hav a preference.

Doctors and all other GP staff are required to keep an information about you confidential, this means that the can't tell anyone anything relating to your appointments o medical history.

Speaking to a GP

You can visit or speak to a GP at any age, and you don't alway have to bring a parent or carer if you don't want to. Althoug if you are under the age of 16, a doctor may need consen from a parent or carer to commence certain treatments suc as prescribed medication.

People over the age of 16 can consent to their ow treatment, this means that they can make decisions abou their own healthcare.

A doctor or nurse might ask you if you want a chaperon this is someone who can sit in the room with you to mak you feel more comfortable. You can request a chaperon when you book your appointment too.

GP's may ask you a range of questions about your problem this is just so that they can find out more about what you'v been experiencing and think about how they can help.

You can ask a GP any questions during your appointment a well, if you're worried that you might forget something, tr making a list beforehand.

10 May 2023

www.healthforteens.co.uk

Consent to treatment

People aged 16 or over are entitled to consent to their own treatment. This can only be overruled in exceptional circumstances.

Like adults, young people (aged 16 or 17) are presumed to have sufficient capacity to decide on their own medical treatment, unless there's significant evidence to suggest otherwise.

Children under the age of 16 can consent to their own treatment if they're believed to have enough intelligence, competence and understanding to fully appreciate what's involved in their treatment. This is known as being Gillick competent.

Otherwise, someone with parental responsibility can consent for them.

This could be:

- the child's mother or father
- the child's legally appointed guardian
- a person with a residence order concerning the child
- a local authority designated to care for the child
- a local authority or person with an emergency protection order for the child

Parental responsibility

A person with parental responsibility must have the capacity to give consent.

If a parent refuses to give consent to a particular treatment, this decision can be overruled by the courts if treatment is thought to be in the best interests of the child.

By law, healthcare professionals only need one person with parental responsibility to give consent for them to provide treatment.

In cases where one parent disagrees with the treatment, doctors are often unwilling to go against their wishes and will try to gain agreement.

If agreement about a particular treatment or what's in the child's best interests cannot be reached, the courts can make a decision.

In an emergency, where treatment is vital and waiting for parental consent would place the child at risk, treatment can proceed without consent.

When consent can be overruled

If a young person refuses treatment, which may lead to their death or a severe permanent injury, their decision can be overruled by the Court of Protection.

This is the legal body that oversees the operation of the Mental Capacity Act.

8 December 2022

www.healthforteens.co.uk

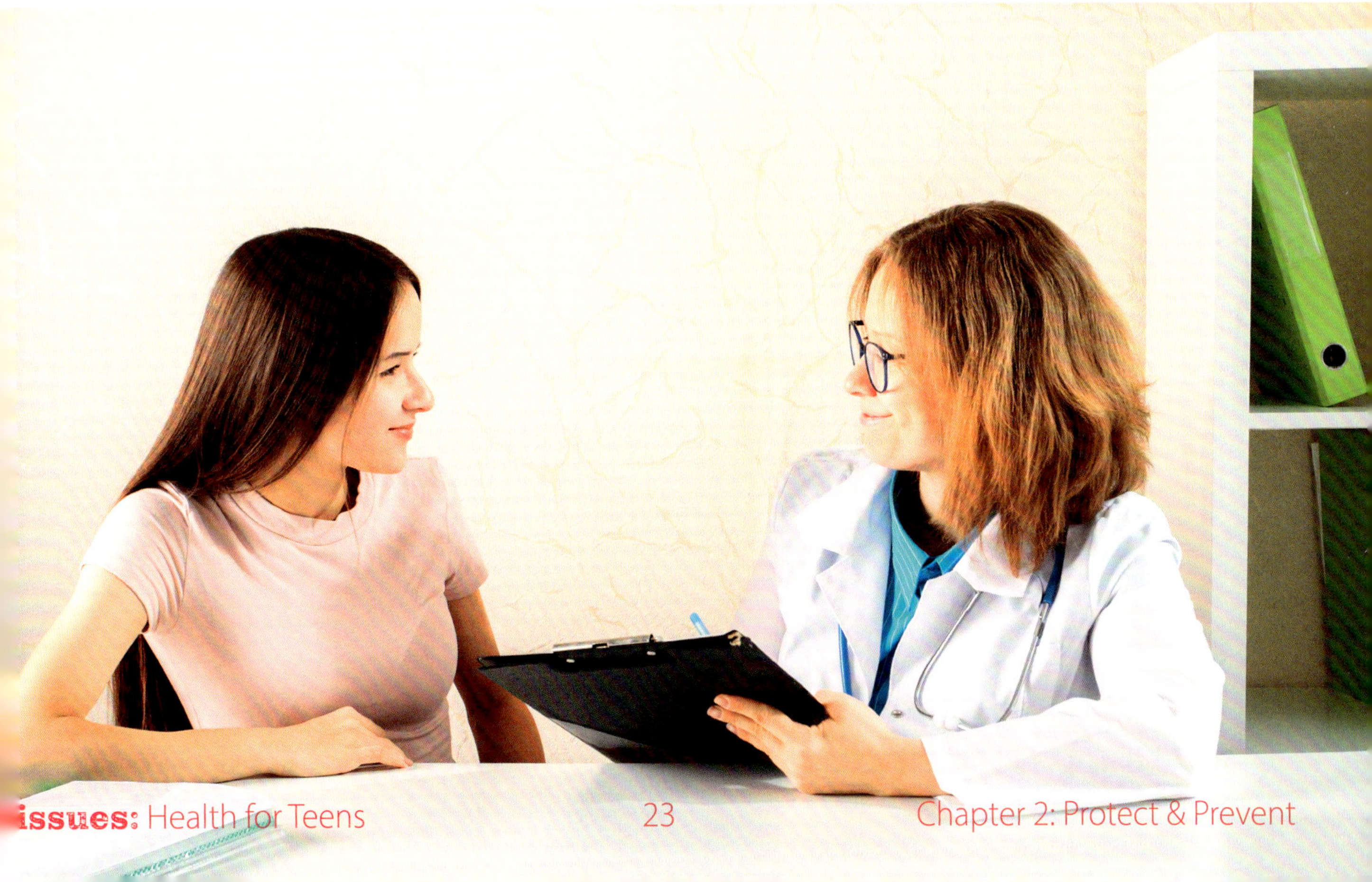

Gillick competency

Gillick competency allows healthcare professionals to decide whether a young person is able to make their own treatment decisions without needing their, or their parent's/carer's involvement

What does Gillick competence mean?

The term 'Gillick competence' was named after Victoria Gillick. She began a legal battle because she didn't want doctors to give the pill to children under 16 without their parents' permission.

In 1985, the judged ruled against her. They decided that doctors and nurses can provide contraception to children under 16 without telling their parents.

One of the judges on the case, Lord Fraser, created some guidelines. These guidelines said that a young person can be provided with contraceptive care if they:

- Are likely to be at risk of being hurt physically or mentally if they don't get the care they request
- Are considered by the doctor or nurse to be 'competent' to consent
- Can't be persuaded to involve a parent or carer in their decision.

Doctors/nurses have to decide if it is in the young person's best interest to get the treatment they ask for and that they would likely continue having sex even without the contraception they ask for.

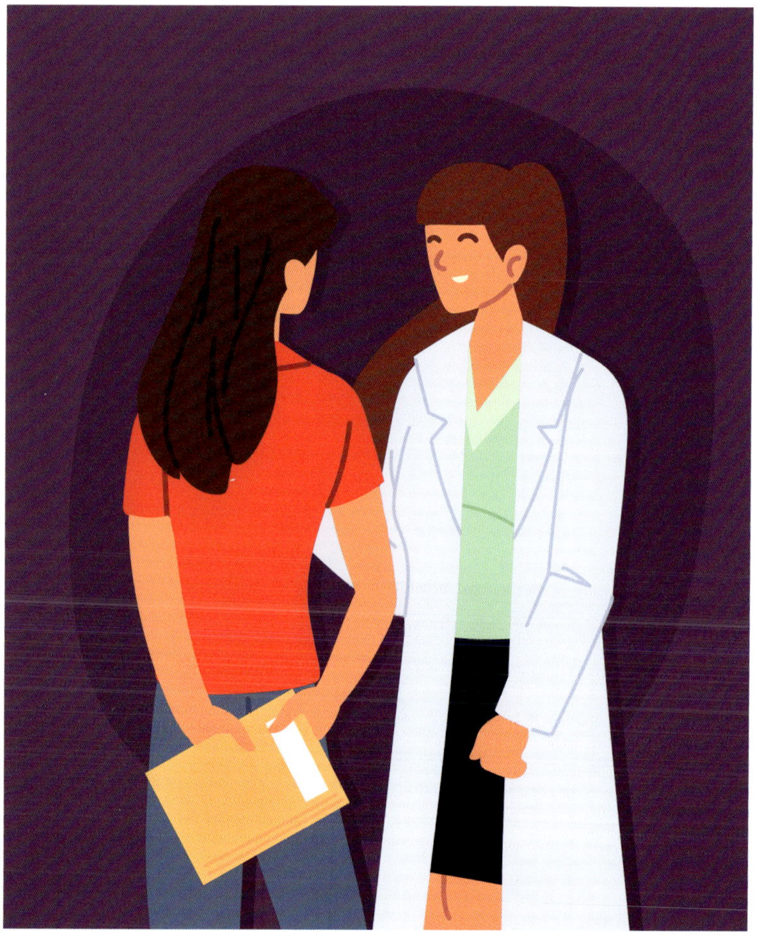

Being 'competent' means:

- Being able to talk through decisions
- Being able to understand and show an understanding of the information that the doctor/nurse has given them about the treatment, including any risks or side effects
- Having the maturity to understand the full impact of their choice

Is Gillick competence just about contraception?

Although the original court case was about contraception for under 16s, the Department of Health later said that the same rules apply to giving abortion care and care for sexually transmitted infections (STIs).

Doctors and nurses use 'Gillick competence' in all areas of health and social care. It is used to check if a young person can make their own decisions about their health or care when:

- They disagree with their parent or carer about the treatment they need
- They don't want to or can't involve a parent or carer
- They want to keep their treatment and situation confidential

Who decides if a young person is competent to consent?

If a young person under 16 wants treatment without their parents' or carers' consent, it is the job and legal duty of the healthcare professional to decide if they are 'competent'. They will do this by:

- Asking the young person questions about the treatment and why they need it
- Or asking for them to explain why they are choosing to refuse a recommended treatment
- Checking the young person's understanding of information they are given
- Finding out what they understand about the treatment, including any risks or side effects of having or not having the treatment
- Discussing any other options they should consider
- Making sure it is the young person's choice and they haven't been persuaded/coerced or forced against their will

- Making sure the young person understands how to use any medication effectively. For example, with contraception they will make sure the young person understands how to use a condom safely, how and when to take their pill, or if they are having an injection that they will need to get it renewed every three months.

Some decisions are more complicated or riskier than others. This means that a young person may be considered 'competent' to make some decisions, for example taking the pill to prevent pregnancy, but not for more complex decisions, like joining a clinical trial of a new cancer drug.

Why is it important for young people to be able to make their own decisions?

It is really important that young people can make their own decisions, especially if involving their parents might be a problem. This might happen if the parents are unhelpful or forceful about treatment choices or if sharing information (like the young person being sexually active) could make them unsafe at home.

Allowing young people to make their own decisions isn't just about safeguarding and keeping them safe; it's also about their rights and autonomy. The United Nations Convention on the Rights of the Child recognises that as children and young people grow and mature, they should have increasing rights to make decisions about things affecting their lives.

Since young people mature and understand things at different rates, each young person is assessed for competence on an individual basis.

Why do doctors/nurses have to 'persuade' a young person to involve a parent or carer?

Parents/carers can be a great source of information, advice and support for their children. In most cases, if a parent knows what's going on in their child's life it can help keep them safe. The younger someone is the most likely they are to benefit from involving their parent/carer.

Doctors/nurses aim to encourage rather than persuade the young person as some parents and carers are not supportive. Involving these parents in these decisions may be harmful or put the young person at risk. The healthcare professional will help the young person weigh up the risks and benefits (pros and cons) of talking to a parent/carer.

If the young person is competent to make their own decision and talking to a parent/carer isn't needed to keep them safe, the doctor/nurse will let the young person make their decision. However, they might suggest talking to the parent/carer with the young person as this can be helpful.

What kind of harm could happen if a young person doesn't get the treatment they ask for?

Here are two examples:

- If a young person wants treatment to stop smoking or drinking alcohol, refusing this treatment could mean they continue doing things that harm their health.
- If a young person is sexually active or is planning to be, not giving them contraception puts them at risk of an unintended pregnancy.

Are there any situations where a young person can't make a decision for themselves?

The most important thing is keeping young people safe and well. In a situation where a young person's choice (i.e., to choose a treatment or refuse a treatment) would put them at extreme risk of harm then their decision can sometimes be overruled by a healthcare professional or a parent/carer.

If a young person isn't Gillick competent do their parents have to be told they asked for treatment?

A young person has the right to confidentiality in healthcare even if they are not mature enough to make treatment decisions. If a young person asked for treatment and it was refused, they could then choose to involve a parent/carer to try to get the treatment they want.

Are healthcare discussions always confidential?

A child's safety and wellbeing is the top priority. Healthcare professionals know that some children and young people are sexually active not by choice, but as a result of abuse, coercion or exploitation.

They may be concerned about a young person because of something they have said about their relationship or partner, or because they have often asked for emergency contraception, have had repeated STIs or have become pregnant (more than once).

If a healthcare professional has to break confidentiality and tell someone, they would pass on the information to a safeguarding professional within their own organisation or in the local authority. The young person should be told about any reports being made and any actions taken.

By law someone under 13 cannot consent to sex. This means if anyone is sexually active under 13, they are considered to be at risk of harm and their case would be discussed by child protection experts for further action.

The above information is reprinted with kind permission from Brook Young People.

www.brook.org.uk

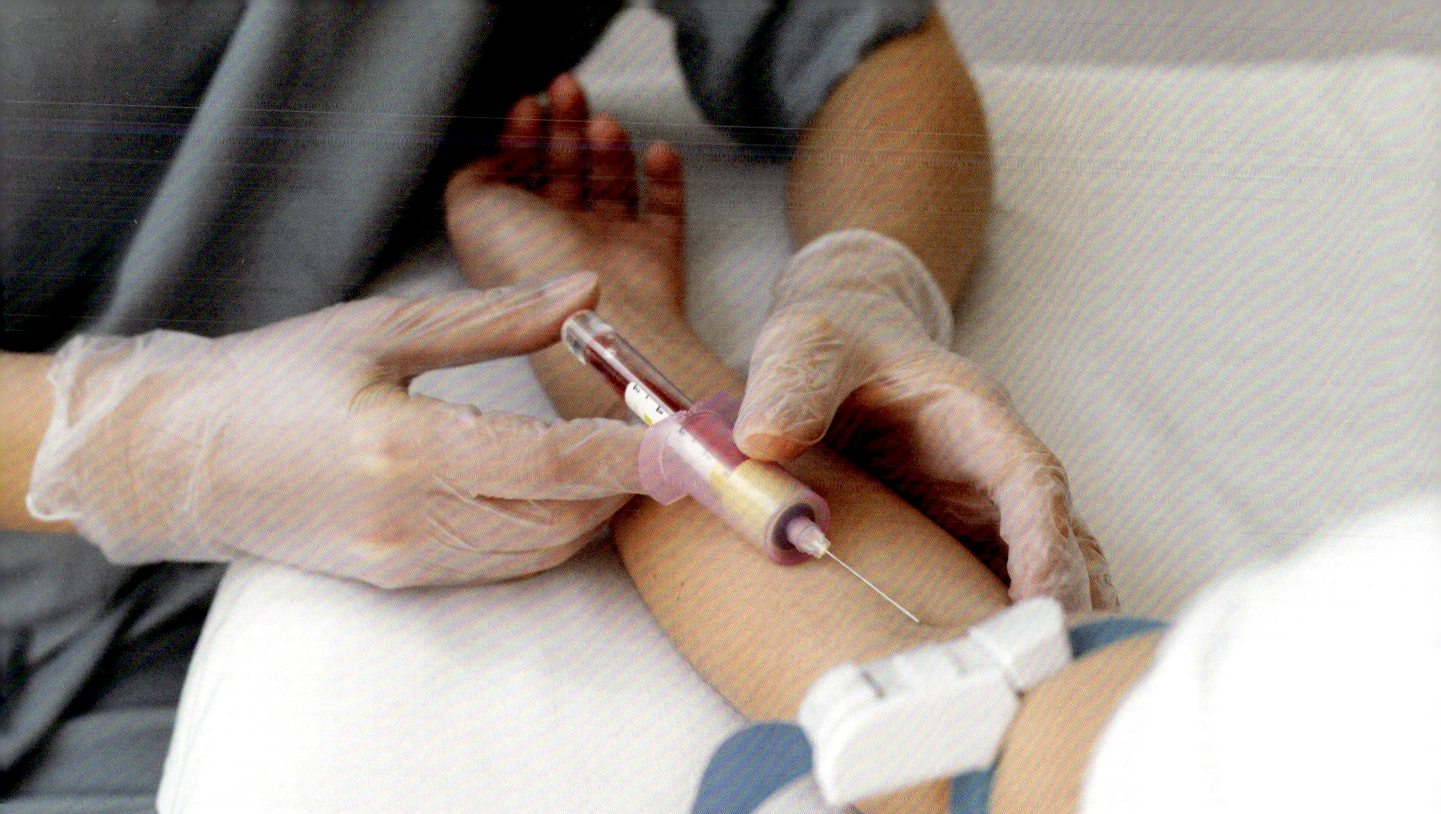

What happens when you go for a blood test?

Hearing you need a blood test can sound scary. Maybe you imagine a giant needle or feel nervous about fainting. The truth is, blood tests are quick, safe and something healthcare staff do every single day. Understanding what actually happens can make the whole thing feel much less stressful.

Why do we need blood tests?

Blood carries a lot of information about how your body is working. Doctors often ask for blood tests to:

- Spot illnesses such as infections, diabetes or anaemia
- Check things like iron, vitamin levels or cholesterol
- Monitor how well treatments are working
- Get an overall picture of your health

It's a simple way of getting answers without any guesswork.

Before the test

Sometimes you'll just be told to come in, while other times you'll book an appointment. Depending on the type of test, you might be asked to avoid food for a few hours (this is called fasting). Drinking water helps keep your veins easier to find. Unless you've been told to fast before the test, have a small snack beforehand.

It's normal to feel anxious, but remember: nurses and phlebotomists (the people trained to take blood) do this all the time. Wearing a short-sleeved top makes the process easier, and you can always ask questions if you're worried.

During the test

You'll usually sit in a special chair with an armrest. The nurs will put a strap called a tourniquet around your arm so th veins are easier to see. The skin is cleaned with a wipe, anc then a small needle goes into the vein.

The first moment might feel like a quick scratch or pinch After that, you'll just notice some pressure as the blooc flows into small tubes. Most tests only take a minute or twc When it's done, the needle comes out and you'll get a cottor pad or plaster on the spot.

After the test

Your arm might feel a bit tender or bruised afterwards - that's completely normal. Try not to do heavy lifting wit that arm for a few hours. If you feel light-headed, sit dow until it passes. Drinking water and having a snack can alsc help, especially if you had to fast.

The blood sample is sent to a lab where it's tested. Result usually go back to your doctor in a few days, depending o the type of test.

Clear answers through a simple process

Blood tests aren't the most fun thing in the world, bu they're nothing to fear. They're quick, safe and give doctor really useful information about what's happening insid your body. The next time you need one, remember – it's jus a small moment that could make a big difference to you health.

Can I donate blood and how do I do it? Urgent call for donors amid low stocks

There is also a 'critical' need for more donors who have the so-called universal blood type – O negative blood.

By Rebecca Whittaker

The NHS needs 200,000 more regular blood donors to sustain a safe and sufficient supply.

Low blood stocks in 2024 prompted an 'amber alert', but blood stocks have remained low ever since.

NHS Blood and Transplant (NHSBT) is now urging more people to donate to avoid a 'red alert', which is a critical situation where public safety is threatened.

It described the past year as 'challenging' for blood stocks, noting that just under 800,000 people are supporting the entire blood supply in England.

How do I donate blood?

The whole process of giving blood takes just one hour. When arriving at a blood donation centre, you are asked to complete a safety check to make sure you can give blood.

You will be given 500ml of fluid to drink – drinking this will help the body maintain blood pressure, prevent dizziness and help the body replenish the donated blood.

Then, to ensure it is safe to donate blood, medics will confirm your identity and information in your health check. In some cases, a registered nurse will follow up.

A drop of blood from your finger is then checked for iron levels. If these levels are too low, the appointment will be rescheduled.

Those able to donate will be seated in the waiting area before being called to a donation chair.

Here, a cuff will be placed on your arm to maintain a small amount of pressure during the donation before a suitable vein is found and the area is cleaned.

Then, a needle will be inserted into your arm to collect your blood into a blood bag, which has your unique donor number on it.

A scale weighs the blood and stops when you have donated 470ml - that's just under a pint.

The needle is then removed from your arm, and a dressing is applied.

The NHS says the process of giving blood should not hurt and should only take about 10 minutes.

Who can donate blood?

Although more donors are needed, there are some health, travel and lifestyle reasons that may stop you from donating blood.

Donors need to be fit and well, aged between 17 and 65, weigh between 7 stone 12 lbs (50kg) and 25 stone (158kg) and have suitable veins.

However, you can't donate blood if you have cancer, some heart conditions, have tested positive for HIV or are a hepatitis B or C carrier.

If you have received blood platelets, plasma or any other blood products after January 1980, or if you have injected non-prescribed drugs including body-building and injectable tanning agents, you also cannot donate.

If you've had anal sex with a new partner in the last three months you may have to postpone your donation.

If you feel unwell, are pregnant or have had a baby in the last six months, have had a tattoo or piercing, or have recently travelled to certain countries outside the UK, you may also have to wait before you can donate blood.

Where can I donate blood?

There are thousands of blood donation venues across England, some are permanent and others are pop-ups.

Church halls, sports centres, mosques, football stadiums and hotels are all used as pop-up venues.

To check where your closest one is, visit the Give Blood website.

You will need to book an appointment ahead of your donation which can be done online as soon as you have signed up as a blood donor.

What type of blood is needed?

There is a 'critical' need for more donors who have the so-called universal blood type, O negative blood, which is needed for treatment in emergencies.

The NHS said there is also a need for more Black donors, who are more likely to have specific blood types which can help treat people with sickle cell disease.

9 June 2025

Design a 'Donate Blood' poster

Design a poster encouraging people to donate blood. Create a catchy slogan and use engaging images.

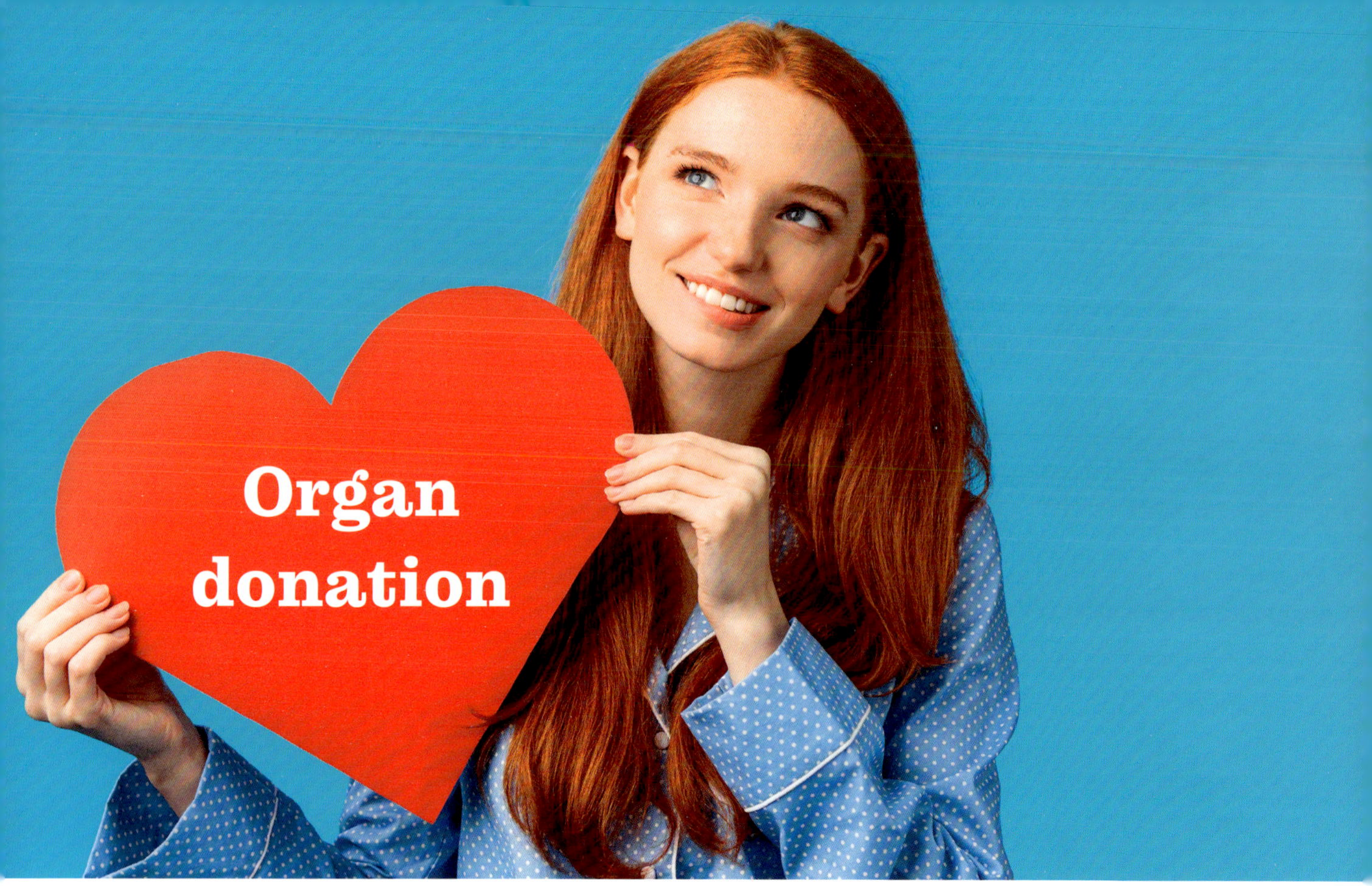

Organ donation

Organ donation is when an organ is given to save or improve the life of someone else. There are many different reasons why someone might desperately need an organ donation to survive. This might be due to a condition they were born with or due to a medical problem they developed later in life.

- In the UK there are over 6,000 people waiting for a transplant
- Three people die everyday in the UK due to lack of available organs.
- One organ donor can save up to nine lives

What is organ donation?

The majority of organs are donated after a person has died (deceased organ donation) but some organs such as kidneys can be donated when a person is alive (living donation). Unless specified the information below is about donation after a person has died.

One organ donor can help up to nine people by donating their organs and many more by donating tissue.

Which organs can be donated

The most commonly transplanted organs are:

- Kidney
- Heart
- Lung
- Pancreas
- Small bowel

There are also many tissues that can be donated such as:

- Cornea
- Heart valves
- Bone

When you join the organ donor register you can choose which organs and tissues you would and wouldn't want to donate.

Who can be an organ donor?

Anyone is able to join the organ donor register. It is important to tell your family and loved ones when you join the register so that they know your wishes.

Can children join the register?

There are no age restrictions on joining the organ donor register but those under 18 need parental consent. Organ transplants are needed by people of all ages and the organ has to be an appropriate size. Therefore donors of all ages are needed.

Is there an upper age limit?

There is no upper age limit. The health of your organs rather than your age is assessed to determine suitability at the time of donation.

What if I have a medical condition?

There is no medical condition that would prevent you from joining the register. The suitability of your organs for donation would be decided by specialist doctors at the time of donation.

Does everyone who registers as an organ donor end up donating?

No. A person has to die in hospital in specific circumstances for their organs to be suitable for donation. This means the majority of people who register as an organ donor are not able to donate their organs when they die. However, tissue donation is often possible even when organ donation is not.

Why ethnicity matters in organ donations:

We need more organ donors from all ethnic backgrounds; however, there is a particular shortage of organs from people of Black and Asian backgrounds in the UK. This means people from Black and Asian backgrounds wait longer for an organ transplant and are more likely to die waiting. Organs have to be matched as well as possible between the donor and recipient. People are most likely to be a close match to someone of their own ethnicity.

Donation rates are currently lower amongst people of Black and Asian backgrounds. Certain conditions that increase the risk of needing a transplant are also more common amongst people of Black and Asian ethnicity.

Law change to opt out of organ donation

Across the UK, there has been a change in the law to an 'opt out' system of presumed consent. This means that everyone is assumed to consent to being an organ donor unless they have opted out by registering that they do not want to be an organ donor.

The opt out law does not apply to people in excluded groups. These are:

- Anyone under the age of 18 (16 in Scotland)
- Those who lack the capacity to understand the law change, make or register their decision
- Those who have been living in the UK for less than one year before they die.

Under the new law families will still be consulted and organ donation will only go ahead if the family are in agreement.

Each part of the UK has its own law on this but key points above apply in England, Scotland, Wales and Northern Ireland. For further details on specifics of the laws in each region see the NHSBT website.

Do I still have a choice?

Yes – Everyone still has a choice in whether or not to be an organ donor.

Do I still need to register a decision?

Yes – You should still register your decision whether or not you want to be an organ donor. It is also very important to tell your family of your decision. This is because your family would be consulted before you become an organ donor and donation will only go ahead if they are in agreement. If you have registered a clear preference and told them of your wishes it is much easier for them to make the decision that you would have wanted. The consent rate from families is only 66% but it is much higher if people have registered a preference to donate and told their family of their wishes.

Will the change in the law increase the number of people who donate?

Opt out systems in other countries have shown that changing the law is not always enough to improve organ donation rates. Instead a change in attitudes is needed. Therefore, there is a clear need for an increase in education about the importance of organ donation and why discussions with friends and family are vital to your decision being respected.

Organ donation and religion

It is a personal decision whether or not you want to donate your organs and how this fits in with your faith and beliefs. There are people from all major religions who decide to donate their organs, however, there are also people from a range of religious backgrounds who do not feel donation fits with their beliefs. If you are unsure whether or not organ donation is compatible with your beliefs, speak to an advisor from your religion. There are also useful resources on the NHSBT website.

Types of donations

Deceased donation

Deceased organ donation is when a person donates their organs after they have died. The above information all relates to deceased donation.

Altruistic donation

A person can donate a kidney or a part of their liver to another person while they are still alive. Most often this is a donation to a loved one but some people also donate an organ to someone they do not know – this is known as altruistic donation.

You can live a normal and healthy life with only one kidney. Prior to donation your health would be checked to ensure that donating a kidney would not have any adverse effect on your health. You would also have to be checked to see if your organs are compatible with the person you want to donate to.

There is a lot more information about living donation on the NHSBT website.

www.wearedonors.co.uk

Everything you need to know about organ donation

Choosing to be an organ donor means leaving a legacy that transforms the lives of others.

Sharing your choice with family and friends is very important, but can sometimes prove tricky because there are many myths and mistaken beliefs about organ donation which hinder discussion and conversation.

Myths and misunderstanding

The truth behind six common organ donation myths.

Myth: When you decide to be a donor, medical teams can use whichever organs they want.

Fact: You can select the organs you want to donate. If you have decided to be a donor, you can visit the NHS donor website and select the organs you want to donate and the ones you don't. At present, donate-able organs include heart, lungs, kidney, liver, small bowel, pancreas and tissue donations which include bone, tendons, corneas and arteries.

Myth: Only BAME (Black, Asian, Middle Eastern) donor organs are suitable for recipients of the same ethnicity.

Fact: It has more to do with blood types. A donated organ from someone within the same blood group is usually more successful, and some blood groups are particular to people with a BAME heritage. In the UK, people with a BAME heritage are less likely to be registered donors, so there's a shortage of suitable organs for people with certain blood types.

Myth: My religion doesn't allow organ donation.

Fact: The major religions endorse organ donation. In the UK, organ donation is consistent with the beliefs of most major religions including Christianity, Islam, Hinduism, Buddhism and most branches of Judaism. However, if you feel it goes against your beliefs, then talk to your local spiritual leader, who can help inform your choice.

Myth: If you're a registered donor and critically ill, medical teams don't try as hard to save you, because they can use your organs to save many more people.

Fact: Your medical team will always be focused on saving your life. In such a crisis, medical teams are totally focused on saving your life and they have a duty of care to you. Your survival and recovery is paramount, not the saving of somebody else's life by removing your organs for them.

Myth: Surgeons can remove your organs before you're actually dead.

Fact: Organs are only removed from people who are clinically brain dead. Organs are removed from donors who are clinically brain dead, in that their brain will never reawaken or be able to sustain life once taken off life support. However, to optimise the quality of organs that can be donated, their circulatory system is kept functioning via a life-support machine until the organs are ready for removal.

Myth: Rich and famous people go to the top of the transplant list when they need a new organ and can even buy them.

Fact: Everybody has to wait for their turn. Celebrity and financial status is not a consideration in organ allocation and they are treated just the same as everybody else. Plus, trafficking and the sale of organs is illegal. When we do hear about celebrities receiving transplants, it may seem that they've been prioritised, but this is usually due to the wide reporting across news networks.

www.livelifegivelife.org.uk

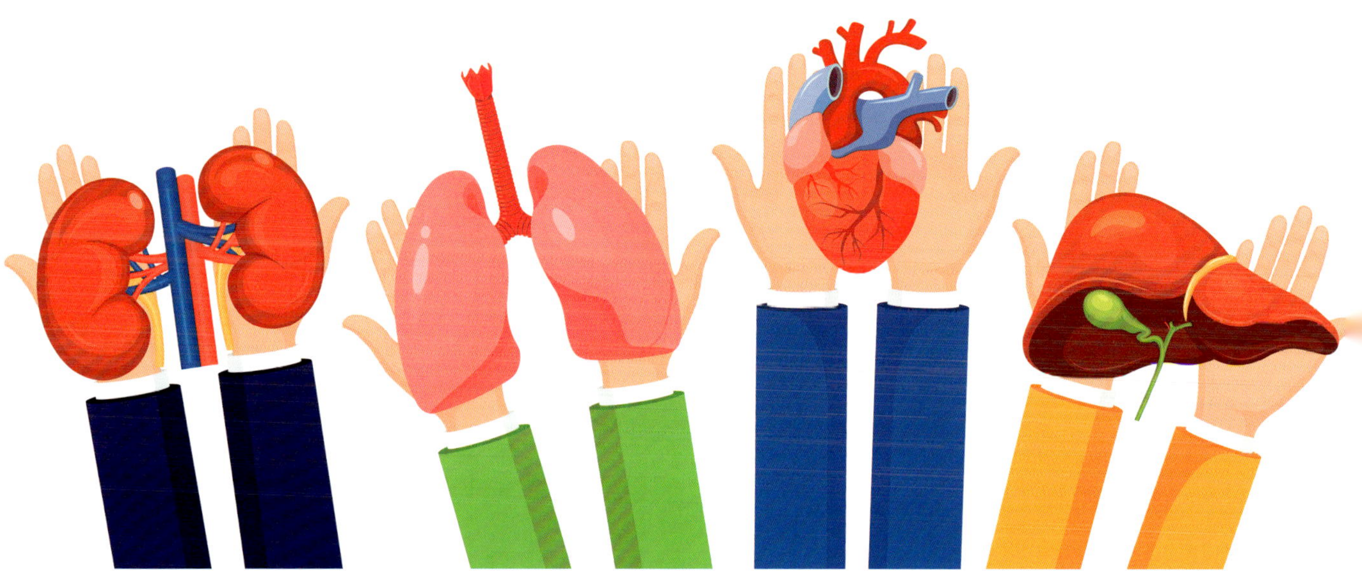

What is self-care?

When people talk about self-care, it can sound like just another trend or a buzzword you see online. But self-care is really about the everyday choices you make to keep your body and mind in a good place. It's not about spending loads of money or creating some perfect routine – it's about knowing what helps you feel calmer, stronger, and ready to deal with life's ups and downs.

Being a teenager means dealing with schoolwork, friendships, family life, and constant online noise. Some days you might feel on top of everything, and other days it might feel like too much. Self-care is not about ignoring your problems – it's about giving yourself the tools and habits to cope better. Think of it as making sure you're charged up, like your phone, so you've got enough energy and focus to handle whatever comes your way.

Why self-care is important for teens

Teenagers often juggle homework, exams, part-time jobs, family expectations, and busy social lives. Add in the fact that your brain and body are still developing, and it's no wonder many teens feel stressed, tired, or overwhelmed. Practising self-care can help by:

- Boosting your energy levels
- Improving focus and concentration
- Supporting good mental health
- Strengthening confidence and resilience
- Helping you feel calmer in stressful situations
- Think of self-care as your personal toolkit. The more you practise, the better prepared you are when things get tough.

Breaking myths about self-care

Some people think self-care is selfish or that you only 'deserve' it once you've worked hard. That's not true. Self-care is about maintenance, like charging your phone battery. You wouldn't wait until your phone is completely dead before plugging it in, so why wait until you're burnt out before looking after yourself?

Taking the first step

Self-care doesn't need to be complicated. Start small – choose one or two habits that feel doable, like drinking more water, getting to bed earlier, or taking five minutes of quiet time before school. Over time, these little actions add up.

Remember: self-care isn't about being perfect. It's about paying attention to what you need and giving yourself permission to take care of your wellbeing.

Self-care is your secret superpower – and the best part is, it's always in your hands.

Switch off sometimes – put your phone down and breathe

Enjoy food that makes you feel energised, not drained

Laugh often – it's the best stress-buster

Focus on sleep (yes, Netflix can wait!)

Chat with friends who hype you up, not drag you down

Activities you love = instant mood boost

Remember movement – dance, skate, kick a ball, whatever's fun

Every small win for your wellbeing matters

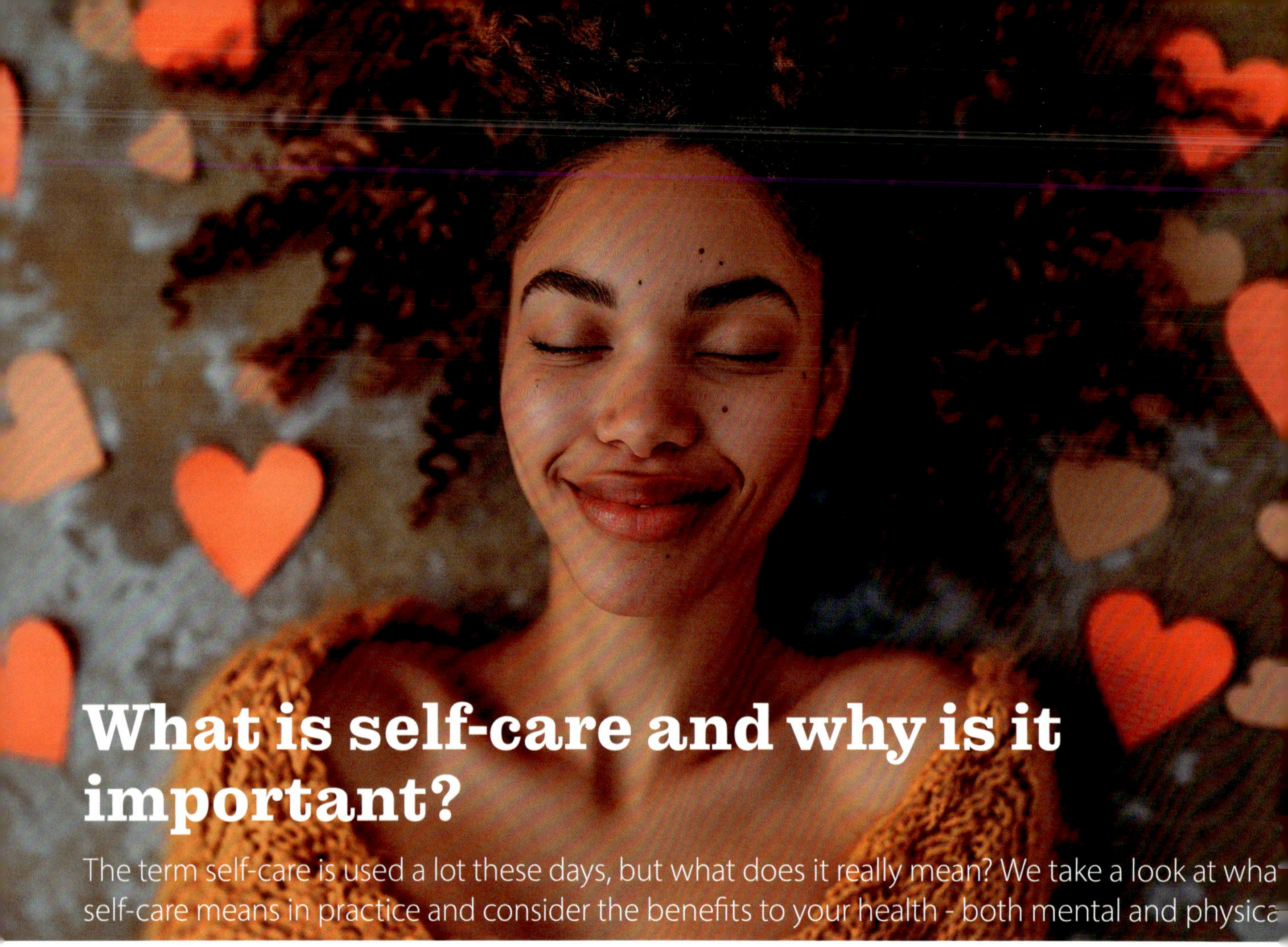

What is self-care and why is it important?

The term self-care is used a lot these days, but what does it really mean? We take a look at wha self-care means in practice and consider the benefits to your health - both mental and physica

What is self-care?

While its popularity in common parlance might be recent, self-care is not a new concept. Nor is it complex, lofty, or exclusive. Self-care is just what it sounds like: taking care of yourself in a way that works for you.

According to the NHS, self-care is the practice of consciously doing things that preserve or improve your mental or physical health.

These days, when people talk about self-care, they are generally talking about the conscious and deliberate choice to do something that looks after you and your wellbeing.

This covers the mental and the physical, and a regime of self-care should improve the way you feel in body and mind. Engaging in acts of self-care or a self-care routine (as many people refer to it), is clinically proven to help reduce or eliminate stress by helping you foster good habits and understand your needs.

Why is self-care important?

Self-care is an important part of living a healthy and happy lifestyle. Looking after yourself both mentally and physically is crucial to taking control of your health.

We lead increasingly busy lives and it can be easy to forget to put yourself first, especially if you have multiple responsibilities and other people to care for. But looking after yourself will make you feel better, and the better you feel, the better you will be in all areas of your life - from wor to relationships.

Self-care doesn't have to involve a huge time commitmen and it doesn't have to cost the earth. It could be taking bath, relaxing with a good book, taking a walk outside o eating your favourite food. It's about making a commitmen to putting yourself first, even just for a while.

> 'Anything you do for yourself that makes you feel better or cared for can be considered self-care.'

What are examples of self-care?

This question is a little harder to answer, because self-car is different for everyone. It's about looking after yourse mentally and physically, and everyone has different needs.

Really, anything you do for yourself that makes you fee better or cared for can be considered self-care. This coul be making sure to floss regularly, it could be taking time t yourself when you need it, it could be getting a new haircu

The term self-care is also used in the medical community t refer to individuals taking charge of their own health. Thi includes everything from making healthy lifestyle choices t taking an active part in managing long-term conditions.

Some people consider meditation a major component c self care. Meditation isn't about transforming yourself c

·our outlook, it is simply about channelling your awareness ·nd developing a better sense of perspective. Learning to neditate takes time, because it is a skill like any other. The act of meditation involves breathwork and focus to be present n the moment and connect with your breathing. Meditation an significantly improve your mental health and become a egular part of your self-care practice.

10 easy ways to practice self-care without spending money

ielf-care doesn't have to cost the earth. Here are some of our top tips for self-care that won't break the bank:

. Get a good night's sleep
. Drink lots of water
. Go for a brisk walk
. Take a relaxing bath
. Say no to something you don't want to do
. Listen to your favourite music
. Watch your favourite film
. Make something healthy yet delicious for dinner
. Make a list of five or more things you like about yourself
0. Spend time with loved ones

What are the benefits of self-care?

elf-care has a number of benefits, most of which are nterlinked. Committing to self-care should improve your vellbeing all round.

ielf-care can improve your physical health

big part of self-care is committing to looking after your ody and becoming more attuned with its needs. Whether 's brushing your teeth, exercising more or getting enough eep each night, part of any programme of self-care should ocus on looking after your physical health. The National ibrary of Medicine has published several studies on the nportance of exercising as a means of self care. These tudies recommend just 30 minutes of walking every day o help boost your mood and improve your health. They tress that small amounts of exercise add up, so don't be iscouraged if you can't do 30 minutes at one time.

elf-care can reduce stress and anxiety

laking time for relaxing activities, such as taking a warm ath, listening to music or practising yoga or meditation, is nother common theme of self-care.

ny activity that makes you feel more relaxed can help to educe symptoms of stress and anxiety and to lift your mood.

> 'Taking time to relax and look after yourself can have a positive impact on the way you see yourself: treating yourself with kindness can make you look upon yourself more kindly.'

Self-care can boost your self-esteem

As well as helping to calm your nerves, taking time to relax and look after yourself can have a positive impact on the way you see yourself: treating yourself with kindness can make you look upon yourself more kindly.

Studies by The National Library of Medicine have found that people with higher self-esteem find it easier to deal with setbacks and are more likely to achieve goals of self-improvement. Self-care can include regular exercise, which helps you stay physically and mentally fit, which can have a positive impact on your self esteem.

Self-care protects your mental health

Making changes to prioritise self-care can help to manage mental health issues and might even prevent them from getting worse.

Of course, self-care is not a substitute for professional help, and you shouldn't feel you have to tackle your problems alone. If your mental health is suffering, you should always talk to someone.

However, if you're looking to improve your mental wellbeing, taking the time to care for yourself both mentally and physically is really important.

The National Institutes of Health has published a self-help, online wellness kit to help you understand best how to look after yourself through a variety of tools.

Self-care can lead to better relationships

It makes sense if you think about it: the happier and healthier you are, the more you can give to a relationship. Not just romantic relationships, but relationships with friends and family, too. If you feel good about yourself, you feel happy and healthy enough to put more attention and time into relationships. Having a solid support network around you is also good for your mental wellbeing, and practising self care can help you foster this network.

This is especially important if you are a parent or carer. It can be so easy to put someone else's needs first, but you must look after your own health too.

The above information is reprinted with kind permission from Circle Health Group.

www.circlehealthgroup.co.uk

Stress snapshot

Draw a 'stress thermometer'. Mark where you are today. Then write one self-care activity that could help you move lower on the scale.

Self-care menu

Create a 'menu' with three quick self-care ideas for the mind (starters), three for the body (mains), and three for relationships (desserts). Illustrate it if you like.

To every kid who's trying

Independence WINNER 11-14 Writing Competition

By Amelie Barbara Dawson, 14

Oxford High School

You are probably going to read this and think it is like every other talk you have heard, but please just listen because this is real. You don't have to be perfect, because I definitely know I'm not perfect. You don't have to have it all figured out. You're still learning, and that means you are meant to make mistakes. Mess up, get things wrong. No matter how much you think you know, there are many things you are yet to know and will learn through your mistakes. That's how you learn.

You don't need to look like anyone else or try to be someone you're not. You are already enough. Your body is not meant to be hated; it is meant to be there to help you every day. Be proud of it. Stop wasting your time worrying about what people think of you. Most of the time, people are too busy worrying about their own insecurities instead of being concerned about yours.

Speak up. I know it feels scary to talk about your feelings, but you need to. You are not 'too emotional' or 'crazy.' You're just human. And you know what? Your parents, yeah, they might understand more than you think. Even if they don't show it perfectly, they care. Let them in. Say something They are there to support you through everything.

And seriously, get off your phone sometimes. Social medi isn't real life. It messes with your head and makes you fee like you're not doing enough. But YOU ARE. You have on life, don't spend it watching other people live theirs. Di you know the average person will spend 12 years staring a their phone screens over their lifespan – yes, shocking!!! G outside. Make something. Try something new.

Right now, you have chances you might not have later. S take them. Join that club, speak your truth, laugh loud, mak art, make friends. Make mistakes. JUST LIVE! You don't nee to wait to be older, or better, or more confident.

This might sound like just another speech, but it is no This is your reminder that you matter. You're not alone, an you're allowed to be free.

And remember it is ok to breathe. To rest. You don't need t be productive all the time; it is okay to take a break, to d nothing. Rest isn't being lazy – it's how you recharge. Don burn yourself out trying to be perfect in school or trying t impress people to fit in. One test, one grade, one momen does not decide your future. What does matter is how yo deal with it through those bad days. How you push throug

Even when you don't believe in yourself – try anyway. Ste forward, even if your voice shakes. Show up, even when it hard. You'll surprise yourself with what you can do. You ar capable of so much more than you think.

And don't forget you are a kid. This is your childhood. It's no supposed to be all stress and pressure. Let yourself be sill Run around. Get messy. Make memories you'll look back o and smile about. This is your time. Live it.

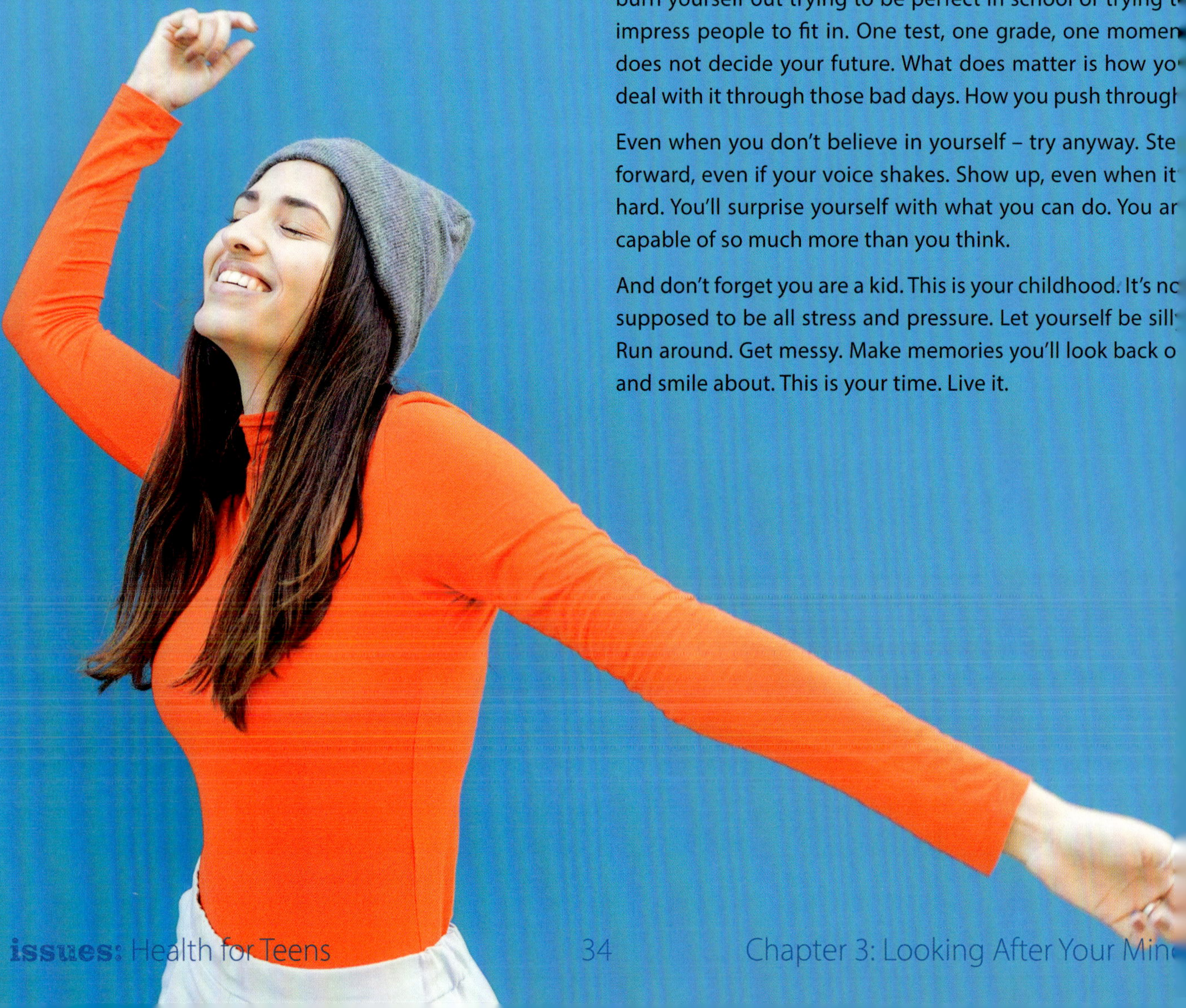

Bees, biscuits, and barely holding it together – my take on self-care

Independence WINNER 15-18 Writing Competition

By Blair Henderson, 17

Stewart's Melville College

Self care. The two words that teachers and motivational posters love throwing around like they've just solved all of life's problems. Feeling stressed? Self-care! Exhausted? Self-care! Forgot to study for that maths test? Don't worry – self-care! The problem is, half the time it feels like nobody really knows what self-care means, or they make it sound like it's all bubble baths and green smoothies. For me, self-care is just doing what I can to get through the week without feeling like I'm falling apart – and, spoiler alert, it's definitely not as glamorous as they make it sound.

Let's talk about what they teach us in school assemblies: 'mindfulness' and 'good routines.' Honestly, I've tried this mindfulness thing. Apparently, it's about focusing on the present moment and breathing deeply, but that's hard to do when your brain is screaming about unfinished homework and the fact that you've run out of clean socks. My version of mindfulness is more like sitting in my room, staring at my computer and eating biscuits until I can pretend my responsibilities don't exist. It's probably not what they had in mind, but it works for me.

And then there's the whole 'get organised' lecture. Teachers make it sound like owning a planner will magically solve everything. I've tried planners. They're fine for the first week, when my handwriting is neat, and everything looks like I've got my life together. By week two, though, it's a disaster. Random notes like 'Buy milk' are scrawled next to 'Essay due,' and by week three, the planner's lost under a pile of books anyway. Some days, self-care is just about admitting that no, I will not be organised today, and yes, I am probably going to wing it.

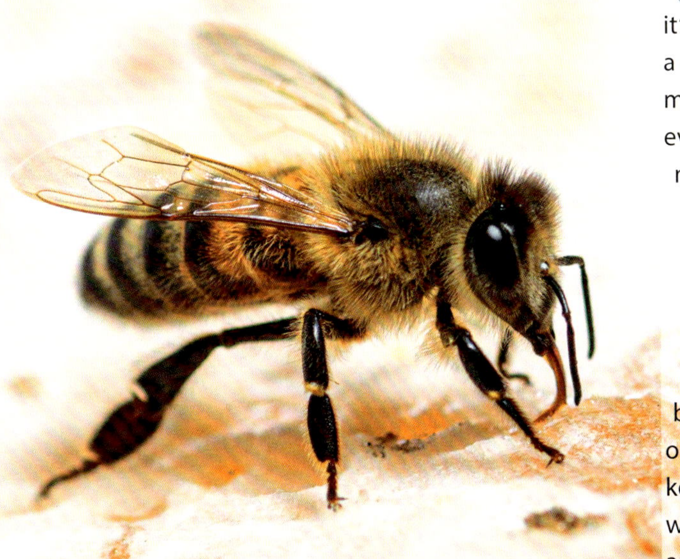

But here's where self-care actually works for me: beekeeping. Yep, you read that right. While most people are out doing yoga or running (been there, hated that), I'm in the garden, looking after my bees. There's something about putting on the suit, hearing the hum of the hive, and watching the bees go about their business that's oddly calming. It's like they know exactly what they're doing, and for that hour or two, I don't have to think about what I'm doing wrong.

Caring for bees is weirdly satisfying. Cleaning the hive, checking for honey, or just watching them buzz around is like hitting a reset button on my brain. Sure, it's not always perfect – like the time I got stung on the nose because I forgot to zip my suit all the way – but even then, it feels like I've done something real, something that matters. Plus, at the end of it all, there's honey, which is basically nature's apology for all the stings.

The thing is, self-care isn't one-size-fits-all. For some people, it's going to the gym or baking sourdough bread. For others, it's about finding the time to read a book or binge-watch a series. For me, it's just about being outside, watching my bees do their thing, and knowing that for a little while, everything is okay. No buzz of schoolwork (pun intended), no pressure to do more or be more – just me, the bees, and the occasional biscuit when I need a snack break.

So yeah, self-care might not look like what they try to sell us in assemblies or in those weird 'wellness' lessons. It's messy, sometimes it involves a lot of trial and error, and occasionally it means getting stung. But that's okay, because it's real. For me, self-care isn't about being perfect or pretending I've got it all together. It's about doing what keeps me grounded – even if that's hanging out with bees while the rest of the world feels like it's going a million miles an hour. And honestly? That's all I need.

Mental health and self-care: a comprehensive guide

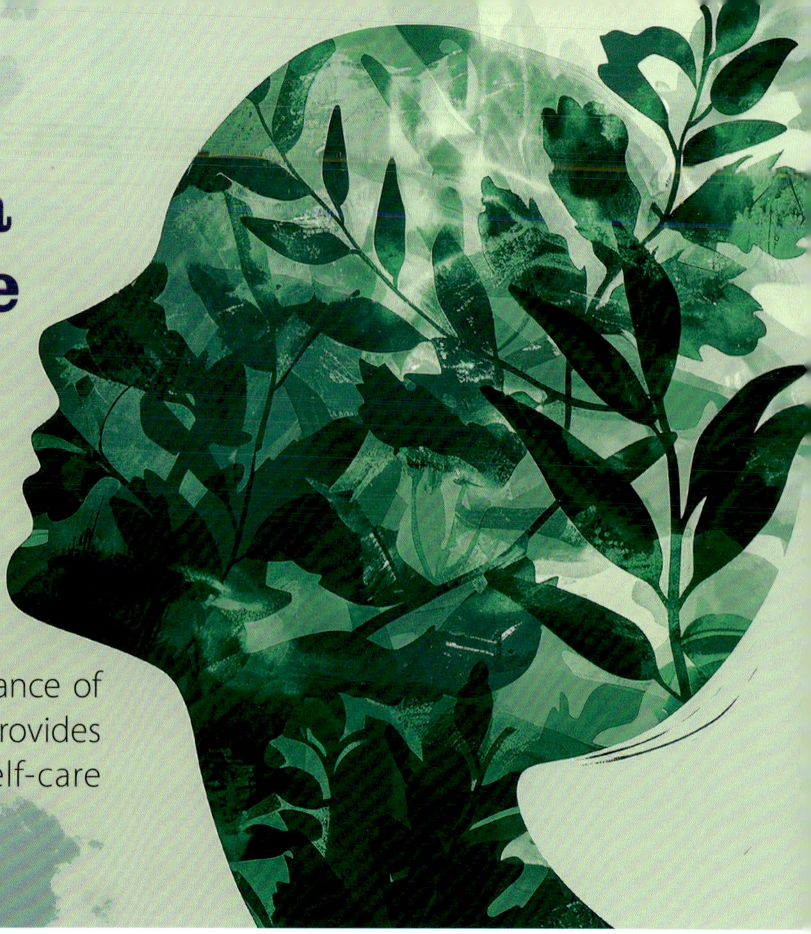

This short guide explores the importance of self-care for good mental health and provides practical tips for implementing self-care strategies.

By David Skinner

Mental health is a cornerstone of overall wellbeing, influencing our thoughts, feelings, and behaviours. It's not merely the absence of mental disorders but a positive state of mind that enables us to cope with life's stresses, realise our potential, and contribute meaningfully to society. Self-care plays a vital role in maintaining mental health. By prioritising self-care, individuals can reduce stress, improve mood, and enhance their quality of life.

The global burden of mental illness

The global prevalence of mental health disorders is significant, with millions of people worldwide affected. Conditions such as depression, anxiety, and bipolar disorder can lead to substantial suffering and impairment. The COVID-19 pandemic further exacerbated these challenges, leading to increased rates of mental health issues.

Understanding mental health

Mental health is a complex interplay of biological, psychological, and social factors. It exists on a spectrum, ranging from optimal wellbeing to severe mental illness.

- Biological factors:
  - Genetic predisposition, neurotransmitter imbalances, and hormonal changes can contribute to mental health conditions.
- Psychological factors:
  - Negative thinking patterns, low self-esteem, and difficulty coping with stress can impact mental health.
- Social factors:
  - Adverse childhood experiences, social isolation and discrimination can increase the risk of mental health problems.

The importance of self-care

Self-care is particularly important in today's fast-paced world, where stress and burnout are common. Practising self-care can reduce stress, improve mood, and enhance overall quality of life. It's a proactive approach to mental health, empowering individuals to manage stress, build resilience, and cultivate a positive outlook.

Key self-care strategies

Physical self-care:

- Regular exercise: Physical activity can boost mood, reduce stress, and improve sleep quality.
- Healthy diet: A balanced diet provides the essential nutrients for optimal brain function.
- Sufficient sleep: Adequate sleep is crucial for cognitive function, emotional regulation, and overall wellbeing.
- Mindful eating: Paying attention to hunger and fullness cues can help regulate eating habits and prevent emotional eating.
- Hydration: Drinking enough water is essential for overall health and wellbeing.

Mental self-care:

- Mindfulness and meditation: These practices can help reduce stress, anxiety, and depression.

970 million
people living with mental disorders

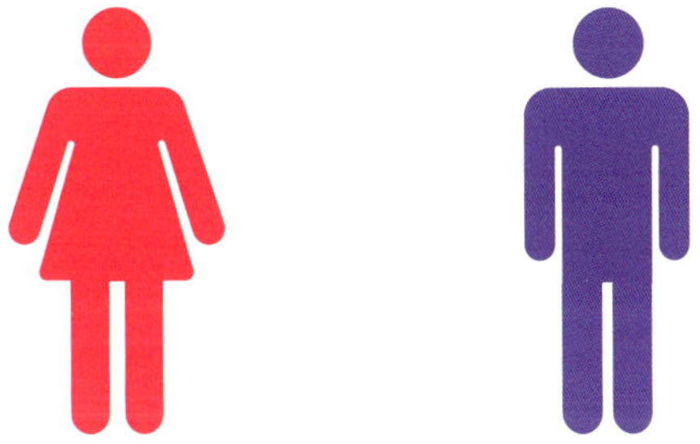

52.4% females

47.6% males

13% of global population is living with mental disorders

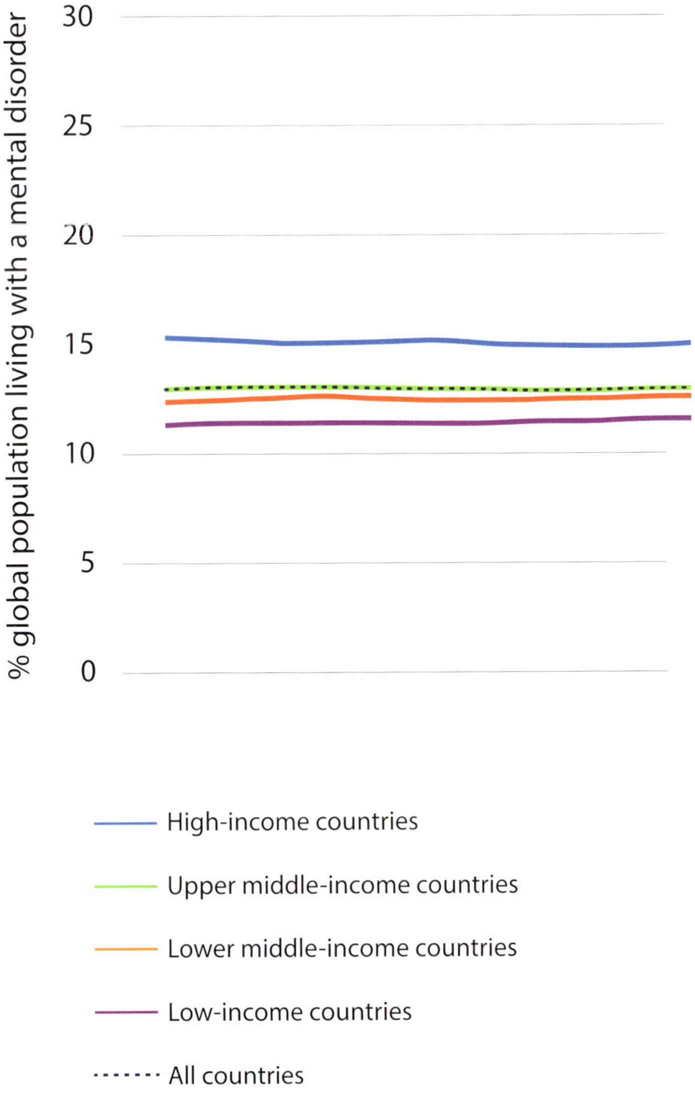

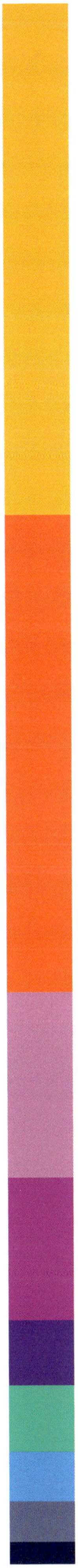

urce: Open Access Government

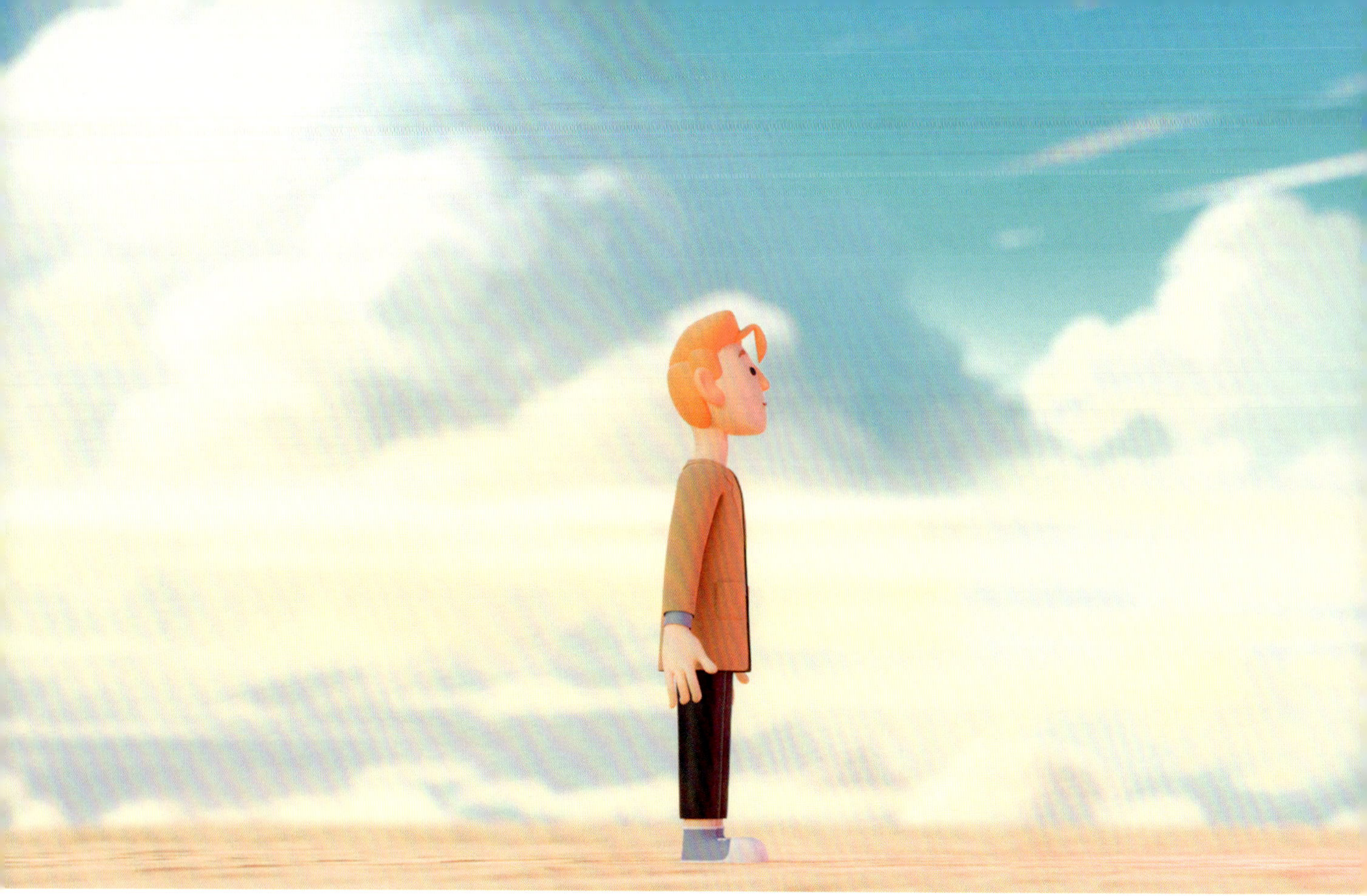

- Cognitive behavioural therapy (CBT): CBT can help individuals identify and challenge negative thought patterns.
- Journaling: Writing about thoughts and feelings can provide emotional release and clarity.
- Digital detox: Taking breaks from technology can reduce stress and improve focus.
- Learning and personal growth: Engaging in activities that stimulate the mind, such as reading, learning new skills, or taking courses.

Emotional self-care:

- Emotional intelligence: Developing emotional intelligence can help individuals understand and manage their emotions.
- Healthy relationships: Strong social connections can provide support and reduce feelings of loneliness.
- Seeking professional help: Therapists and counsellors can provide guidance and support.
- Practising gratitude: Focusing on positive aspects of life can improve overall wellbeing.
- Assertiveness: Learning to communicate effectively and set boundaries can help reduce stress and improve relationships.

Spiritual self-care:

- Spiritual practices: Engaging in religious or spiritual practices can provide comfort and meaning.
- Connecting with nature: Spending time in nature can reduce stress and promote relaxation.
- Engaging in hobbies: Pursuing hobbies and interests can provide joy and fulfilment.
- Practising gratitude: Focusing on positive aspects of life can improve overall wellbeing.

Overcoming barriers to self-care

Numerous barriers can hinder individuals from prioritising self-care. These include:

- Stigma:
  - Negative attitudes and stereotypes associated with mental health can discourage people from seeking help.
- Lack of time:
  - Busy schedules and demanding lifestyles can make it difficult to prioritise self-care.
- Financial constraints:
  - Limited financial resources can restrict access to mental health services and self-care activities.
- Lack of awareness:
- Many people may not recognise the importance of self care or may not know how to practice it effectively.

Strategies for overcoming barriers

To overcome these barriers, consider the following strategies:

- Prioritise self-care:

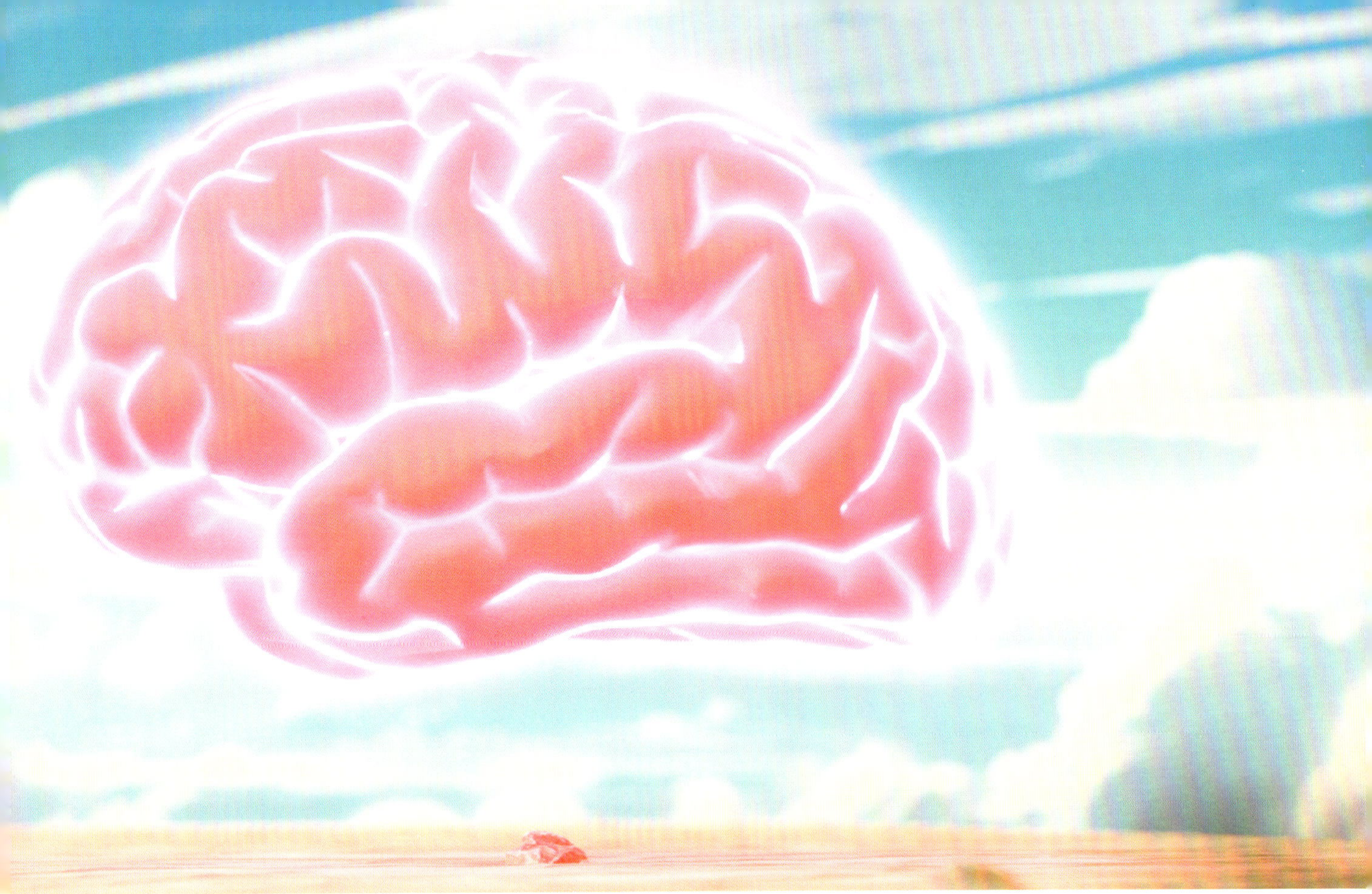

- Make self-care a non-negotiable part of your daily routine.

- Set realistic goals:
  - Start small and gradually increase the frequency and intensity of self-care activities.
- Seek support:
  - Reach out to friends, family, or mental health professionals for support and guidance.
- Challenge stigma:
  - Educate yourself and others about mental health and reduce stigma.
- Practice self-compassion:
  - Be kind to yourself and avoid self-criticism.
- Time management:
  - Effective time management can help you balance your commitments and prioritise self-care.
- Budgeting:
  - Allocate funds for self-care activities, such as therapy, yoga classes, or massages.
- Educate yourself:
  - Learn about mental health and self-care strategies to empower yourself.

Investing in your long-term health and happiness

Prioritising self-care can lead to increased resilience, better relationships, improved productivity, and greater overall life satisfaction. Remember, it's never too late to prioritise your mental health.

By making small changes and incorporating self-care practices into your daily routine, you can experience a significant positive impact on your mental wellbeing.

13 January 2025

Music for your mood

Make a playlist of 5–10 songs that support your mental health. Split it into two sections: (a) calming tracks to relax you, and (b) energising tracks that lift your mood. Write a short note about when you'd listen to each section.

Create a one-week self-care plan

Choose one habit to focus on for the next 7 days (for example: drink more water, go for a short walk, switch your phone off before bed, or write down three positives each evening).

Step 1: Write down your chosen habit.

Step 2: Plan how you'll remind yourself to do it each day (alarm, checklist, sticky note, or a friend to encourage you).

Step 3: At the end of each day, record whether you managed it and how it made you feel.

Step 4: At the end of the week, reflect – was it helpful? Do you want to continue or try a different habit next week?

5 steps to mental wellbeing

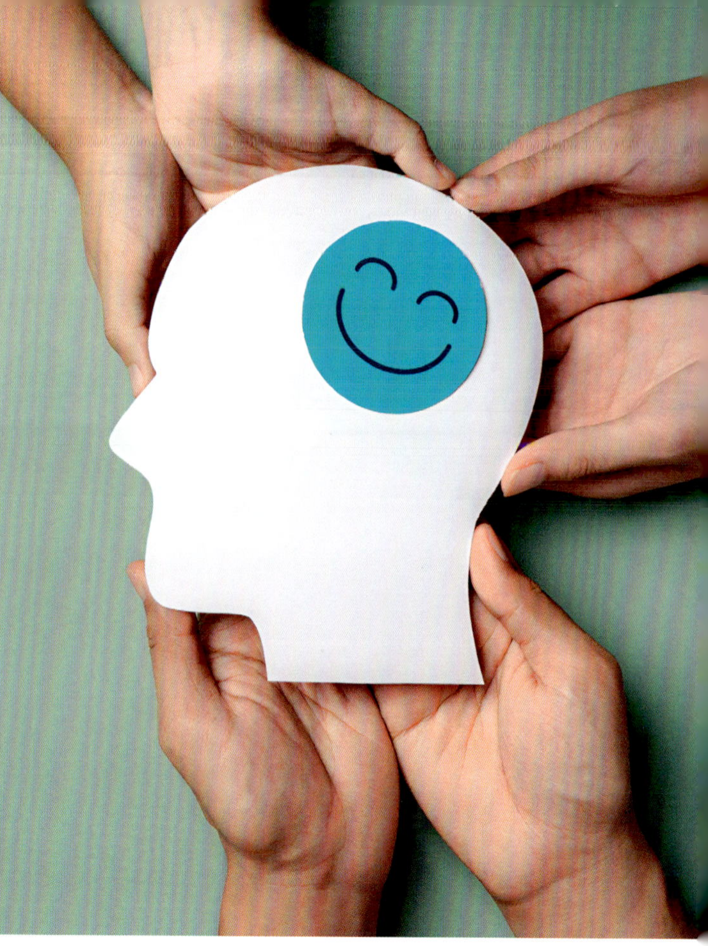

Evidence suggests there are 5 steps you can take to improve your mental health and wellbeing. Trying these things could help you feel more positive and able to get the most out of life.

1. Connect with other people

Good relationships are important for your mental wellbeing. They can:

- help you to build a sense of belonging and self-worth
- give you an opportunity to share positive experiences
- provide emotional support and allow you to support others

There are lots of things you could try to help build stronger and closer relationships:

Do

- ✅ if possible, take time each day to be with your family, for example, try arranging a fixed time to eat dinner together
- ✅ arrange a day out with friends you have not seen for a while
- ✅ try switching off the TV to talk or play a game with your children, friends or family
- ✅ have lunch with a colleague
- ✅ visit a friend or family member who needs support or company
- ✅ volunteer at a local school, hospital or community group. Find out how to volunteer on the GOV.UK website
- ✅ make the most of technology to stay in touch with friends and family. Video-chat apps like Skype and FaceTime are useful, especially if you live far apart

Don't

- ❎ do not rely on technology or social media alone to build relationships. It's easy to get into the habit of only ever texting, messaging or emailing people

2. Be physically active

Being active is not only great for your physical health and fitness. Evidence also shows it can also improve your mental wellbeing by:

- raising your self-esteem
- helping you to set goals or challenges and achieve them
- causing chemical changes in your brain which can help to positively change your mood

Do

- ✅ read about running and aerobic exercises to help get you moving and improve your fitness
- ✅ read about strength and flexibility exercises to increase muscle strength, improve balance and reduce joint pain
- ✅ if you're a wheelchair user, read fitness advice for wheelchair users

Don't

- ❎ do not feel you have to spend hours in a gym. It's best to find activities you enjoy and make them a part of your life

3. Learn new skills

Research shows that learning new skills can also improve your mental wellbeing by:

- boosting self-confidence and raising self-esteem
- helping you to build a sense of purpose
- helping you to connect with others

Even if you feel like you do not have enough time, or you may not need to learn new things, there are lots of different ways to bring learning into your life.

Some of the things you could try include:

Do

- ✅ try learning to cook something new. Find out about eating a healthy, balanced diet
- ✅ try taking on a new responsibility at work, such as mentoring a junior staff member or improving your presentation skills
- ✅ work on a DIY project, such as fixing a broken bike, garden gate or something bigger. There are lots of free video tutorials online
- ✅ consider signing up for a course at a local college. You could try learning a new language or a practical skill such as plumbing
- ✅ try new hobbies that challenge you, such as writing a blog, taking up a new sport or learning to paint

Don't

- ❎ do not feel you have to learn new qualifications or sit exams if this does not interest you. It's best to find activities you enjoy and make them a part of your life

4. Give to others

Research suggests that acts of giving and kindness can help improve your mental wellbeing by:

- creating positive feelings and a sense of reward
- giving you a feeling of purpose and self-worth
- helping you connect with other people

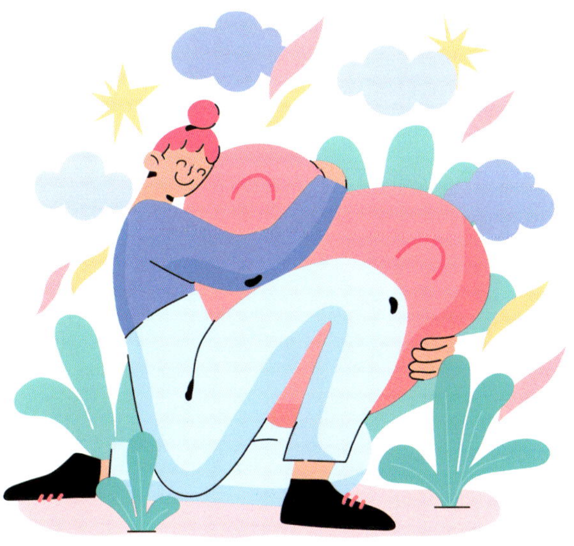

It could be small acts of kindness towards other people, or larger ones like volunteering in your local community.

Some examples of the things you could try include:

- saying thank you to someone for something they have done for you
- asking friends, family or colleagues how they are and really listening to their answer
- spending time with friends or relatives who need support or company
- offering to help someone you know with DIY or a work project
- volunteering in your community, such as helping at a school, hospital or care home

5. Pay attention to the present moment (mindfulness)

Paying more attention to the present moment can improve your mental wellbeing. This includes your thoughts and feelings, your body and the world around you.

Some people call this awareness 'mindfulness'. Mindfulness can help you enjoy life more and understand yourself better. It can positively change the way you feel about life and how you approach challenges.

16 December 2022

www.nhs.uk

Brainstorm race

In pairs, set a timer for 5 minutes. List as many self-care activities as you can think of that cost nothing. After the time is up, share your list with the class and combine them to make a giant 'self-care wall'.

Stress reflection journal

Think about the last time you felt stressed. Write a short description of what happened. Then, list: (a) what triggered your stress, (b) how your body reacted, and (c) how you coped. Finally, note one healthier strategy you could try next time.

Digital detox

Choose one evening this week to go screen-free. No TikTok, no gaming, no scrolling. Instead, do something restful: read, draw, or just sit quietly. The next morning, jot down how you slept and how your mood feels.

Useful Websites

Useful websites

www.brook.org.uk

www.circlehealthgroup.co.uk

www.dentalhealth.org

www.healthforteens.co.uk

www.independent.co.uk

www.livelifegivelife.org.uk

www.nhs.uk

www.openaccessgovernment.org

www.theconversation.com

www.theguardian.com

www.wearedonors.co.uk

www.yougov.com

Acne

A common skin condition where pores become blocked with oil, dead skin, or bacteria, leading to spots, blackheads, or cysts. It often begins in adolescence but can affect people of any age.

Adolescence

The stage of life between childhood and adulthood, usually ages 10–19. Adolescence is marked by changes in the body, emotions, and relationships that shape identity and health.

Adolescent

A young person in the transitional stage between child and adult. Adolescents go through physical, mental, and social changes that prepare them for adult life and independence

Anxiety

A strong feeling of worry, nervousness, or fear. While common before challenges, anxiety can become overwhelming, making everyday tasks, sleep, and social life difficult to manage.

Balanced diet

Eating a variety of foods in the right amounts to provide nutrients such as carbohydrates, protein, fats, vitamins, and minerals. A balanced diet supports growth, energy, and health.

Blood donor

A person who voluntarily gives blood to help others. Donated blood is vital in hospitals for operations, emergencies, and treatments, supporting the survival and recovery of patients

Body image

The way someone thinks and feels about their body's size, shape, and appearance. Body image can influence confidence and self-esteem, and is often shaped by peers, culture, and media.

Body odour

A smell caused when sweat mixes with bacteria on the skin. Body odour is normal but can be reduced through good hygiene, fresh clothes, and the use of deodorants or antiperspirants.

Dental hygiene

The practice of caring for teeth and gums by brushing, flossing, and regular dental check-ups. Good dental hygiene prevents decay and disease and keeps the whole body healthier.

Glossary

)igital detox

\ planned break from using devices such as phones, laptops,)r games consoles. It helps reduce stress, improve focus, ınd reconnect with hobbies, friends, and the offline world.

:ndorphins

\atural chemicals released in the brain that reduce pain ınd boost mood. They are often released during exercise, aughter, or enjoyable activities, helping improve wellbeing.

:xam stress

eelings of worry, fear, or pressure linked to tests. A ıttle stress can help motivation, but too much can harm vellbeing. Strategies such as rest, planning, and breaks can ıelp.

:xercise

\ny physical activity that strengthens the body and upports health, from walking and dancing to sports and ym workouts. Regular exercise improves fitness, mood, and nergy levels.

:itness

'he state of being healthy in body and mind. Fitness often neans strength, stamina, or flexibility, but also includes nental resilience. It improves with exercise, diet, and rest.

;P

hort for General Practitioner – a community doctor who reats a wide range of health issues. GPs provide advice,)rescriptions, and referrals to specialists when needed.

Iormones

:hemical messengers made by glands that travel in the)lood to organs and tissues. They guide growth, puberty, nood, sleep, appetite and energy. Levels naturally change; tress or illness can affect how you feel and function.

Iygiene

'ractices that keep the body and environment clean, such as vashing, handwashing, and hair care. Good hygiene helps revent illness and boosts confidence and wellbeing.

mmune system

'he body's defence system against illness and infection. It ecognises and fights harmful germs and remembers them, ffering protection from future diseases.

/lenstruation

'he monthly process where the womb lining is shed, also alled a period. It is a natural part of the menstrual cycle for eople with female reproductive systems.

/lental health

\ person's emotional, psychological, and social wellbeing. t affects how we think, feel, and act. Good mental health upports relationships, learning, and coping with challenges.

/lindfulness

he practice of focusing attention on the present moment almly and without judgement. It helps reduce stress, nanage emotions, and improve concentration and selfwareness.

NHS

The National Health Service in the UK provides free healthcare to residents. Services include GP visits, hospital care, mental health support, and emergency treatment.

Organ donor

A person who chooses to give their organs or tissues, usually after death, to help save or improve the lives of others. Registration is voluntary but has a life-changing impact.

Peer pressure

Influence from friends, classmates, or social groups to behave in certain ways. It can be positive, such as encouraging healthy choices, or negative, like risky behaviour.

Puberty

The stage when a child's body begins to change into an adult body, with physical changes such as growth, voice change, and menstruation, as well as emotional developments.

Resilience

The ability to recover from challenges, setbacks, or stress. Resilience helps people adapt positively, build confidence, and manage life's ups and downs more effectively.

Self-care

Looking after your physical and mental health through habits such as exercise, relaxation, good food, and rest. Self-care keeps you balanced, energised, and resilient.

Self-compassion

Being kind to yourself in difficult times instead of being overly critical. Self-compassion helps build emotional strength, supports recovery, and promotes a positive mindset.

Self-esteem

How someone feels about themselves and their value. Good self-esteem builds confidence and resilience, while low self-esteem may cause doubt, sadness, or self-criticism.

Skincare

Steps taken to keep skin clean and healthy, such as cleansing, moisturising, and sun protection. Skincare supports confidence and can prevent acne, dryness, or irritation.

Sleep hygiene

Healthy habits that help you sleep well, like keeping a routine, limiting screens before bed, and creating a calm environment. Good sleep hygiene supports focus and wellbeing.

Stress

The body's reaction to pressure or demands. Small amounts can motivate, but too much can harm health. Stress may affect mood, sleep, or focus, and coping strategies can help.

Wellbeing

A broad term covering physical, emotional, and social health. Wellbeing means feeling balanced, connected, and able to cope with life's challenges in positive ways.

Index